The
Healing
Bath

The Healing Bath

Using Essential Oil Therapy
to Balance Body Energy

MILLI D. AUSTIN

Healing Arts Press
Rochester, Vermont

Healing Arts Press
One Park Street
Rochester, Vermont 05767
www.gotoit.com

LIBRARY OF CONGRESS CATALOGING-IN-PUBLICATION DATA
Austin, Milli D.
    The healing bath : using essential oil therapy to balance body
energy / Milli D. Austin.
        p. cm.
    Includes index.
    ISBN 0-89281-632-5
    1. Aromatherapy.   2. Baths—Therapeutic use.   I. Title.
RM666.A68A97   1996
615'.321—dc20   96-21033
                                                           CIP

Printed and bound in Canada

10 9 8 7 6 5 4 3 2 1

Type design and layout by Peri Champine
This book was typeset in New Baskerville Roman

Healing Arts Press is a division of Inner Traditions International

Distributed to the book trade in Canada by Publishers Group West (PGW),
    Toronto, Ontario

Distributed to the health food trade in Canada by Alive Books, Toronto and
    Vancouver

Distributed to the book trade in the United Kingdom by Deep Books,
    London

Distributed to the book trade in Australia by Millennium Books, Newtown,
    N. S. W.

Distributed to the book trade in New Zealand by Tandem Press, Auckland

Distributed to the book trade in South Africa by Alternative Books,
    Ferndale

Table of Contents

A Note to the Reader   vii

Introduction   1

1   Human Subtle Bodies   7

2   The Chakra System and Human Evolution   43

3   Essential Oils and Their Healing Properties   63

4   Apple Cider Vinegar and Gemstones
      in the Bath   74

5   The Bathtub   79

6   Bath Instructions and Formulas   83

7   Instructions and Formulas for Massage   127

    Appendix A: List of Essential Oils   141

    Appendix B: Essential Oil Therapy
      Classes   145

    Appendix C: Resources for Essential Oils   146

A Note to the Reader

Essential Oil Therapy is a spiritual practice that serves to release us from constrictions and in so doing brings forth greater health and happiness through the cleansing and healing of the aura or energy field. It is a therapy that addresses other dimensions of our nature with which many in the Western world are unfamiliar.

The kinds of reactions that may occur as a result of the baths can easily be misunderstood. Markings on the skin, blotches, unusual raised geometric configurations, mild rashes, and, in extreme cases, skin eruptions may occur as the result of anger or fear releases. If they do occur and are painful, get out of the bath immediately and reduce the concentration of essential oils in your next bath. Read and follow the guidelines for taking the baths, as well as the individual bath instructions, which normally minimize these types of responses but do not guarantee that they won't occur. Do not begin

Essential Oil Therapy before reading all the chapters in this book.

This book is intended as an informational guide. The remedies, approaches, and techniques described herein are meant to supplement, and not to be a substitute for, professional medical care or treatment. They should not be used to treat a serious ailment without prior consultation with a qualified health-care professional.

The guidelines and instructions in this book should be carefully followed. If formulas are found to be more powerful than desired, cut the formulas in half and work from there. It is recommended that baths be done under the guidance of an experienced practitioner. People with medical problems, pregnant women, or those who are in poor health or extremely weakened conditions should not do the baths.

This work focuses on healing the subtle, intangible parts of ourselves that directly influence and condition the physical body. While healing at the physical level does take place, this is a result of healing in the energy field.

Introduction

In one way or another everything that has happened to me in this lifetime has culminated in and is reflected in the development of Essential Oil Therapy. I always had a sense of urgency, a need to "complete the mission" yet simultaneously I drew a blank as to what it meant, this sense of mission. Who would have thought that the tools and direction would come from being a businesswoman? That certainly is not the common approach to spiritual creativity. Yet it was my experience in the business world that propelled me onto my spiritual path and eventually led to my becoming an ordained minister.

In 1975 I became public relations director for a worldwide yoga society. During that year I spent time in the Bahamas and traveled the North American continent, writing articles for newspapers, giving radio and television interviews, and assisting in the scheduling and promotion of events. It was a fascinating year, a kaleidoscope of special events, masses of people, famous names, and spiritual teachers.

In the West our primary focus for the treatment of disease has been the physical body. This has been the technique of Western medicine, and it has become deeply ingrained in the public psyche. But by doing this, Western medicine addresses only the physical symptoms of illness and not the underlying spiritual/emotional cause.

Preventive medicine is the foundation of the Eastern approach to good health. It not only sets forth guidelines for regular health practices but also incorporates the recognition of seven bodies, six of which are energy fields that interpenetrate the physical body and extend several feet outward from it. The spiritual nature of humanity, the soul, is included within the art of healing. In fact, it is a central and crucial aspect.

Understanding Essential Oil Therapy is not possible by focusing only on the physical body. The whole human being must be considered when interpreting the effects of essential oils. Otherwise, misconceptions and gaps in understanding will occur.

Through observation and personal experiences at ashrams, I developed the knowledge that allowed me insight into the nature of illness. Many years of intense study and spiritual practices culminated in my development of Essential Oil Therapy.

The energy of an ashram cannot be accurately anticipated, especially by a person who has never visited one. Before my first exposure to an ashram I imagined that it would be an experience of living in a peaceful environment where people would be loving, kind, understanding, and supportive. I did not understand the dynamics of this spiritual energy and the catalytic effects that they have on people.

I had the opportunity to watch these dynamics in action at four ashrams and numerous centers in Canada and the United States. People would come looking for rest and renewal. They would arrive with a hurried and tense energy about them, and their faces mirrored the internal stress. It became easy to spot new arrivals.

After a few days the tension and stress would melt. In an ashram the cathartic and cleansing energies set in place through continual meditation and spiritual practices affect everyone who enters the energy field. People begin to purge their emotional and mental toxins as they become immersed in a less toxic and more light-filled environment. This, combined with meditation, breath work, a healthful diet, and daily yoga exercise, promotes a remarkable cleansing response.

I was completely unprepared for what I perceived to be the irrational, out of control, emotionally overwrought behavior of many guests and of some of the students who were there for the yoga teachers training class.

I, too, took the yoga teachers training class. It was my first assignment. The six-week course culminated in graduation and certification as yoga teachers for all class members who made it through to the end.

My year-long experience was a training ground where I learned to understand the energy dynamics that cause spiritual purging and the acting out that often takes place at the beginning of the purification process. It appeared at times that people were falling apart at the seams. Yet it was all calmly taken in stride by seasoned visitors and staff.

What I learned from this experience was invaluable. It provided an opportunity for me to observe how traumas are pushed down and held in and how little most people are aware of the emotional and mental weight that they carry from day to day.

In yoga there are traditions thousands of years old, practices that are structured to clear and process. No one gets overly concerned if guests or staff members become emotionally overwrought or move through what is commonly called a healing crisis. There were times when I felt that it would have been useful to have counselors, trained therapists, available for those who wanted them, but there is imbued in the yogic approach a deep understanding of human nature. The spiritual practices that have been developed are highly effective. There are disciplines to be followed and daily practices and rituals that serve to stabilize and strengthen one during this internalized journey of self-discovery.

Through personal experience, observation, and interaction with many of these people I learned about the hidden effects of past lives and the way they play out. I learned about purification, the many levels to be explored, and the ways in which people are affected. This opened a whole realm of exploration untouched by my Christian upbringing, and provided many of the answers I had been seeking. For as long as we look to authority figures for all the answers, we never come to know the wisdom of our inner being.

The experience prepared me for the wide range of responses that people have when they take the baths or use the essential oils in various ways. When people had past-life memories or spiritual experiences that didn't fit into Western concepts, their responses paralleled those I had witnessed in the ashrams.

Consequently, the work that I have developed with Essential Oil Therapy brings with it an understanding of the wisdom and strengthening practices of Eastern traditions. At the same time, I always encourage people to seek out other alternative therapies being practiced in the West that will lend needed support and assistance in moving through their journey toward a more conscious lifestyle and accelerated evolution. Counseling, group therapy, Rolfing, massage, acupuncture, breath work, zero balancing, Reiki, Trager, meditation, prayer, craniosacral work, reading, diet, herbs—all are beneficial. In my private practice I frequently advise specific programs that incorporate other therapies. No one therapy is a complete therapy. We are multifaceted, multidimensional beings, and we require a variety of modalities to meet our needs.

The word *evolution* as used in this book means a natural process of unfoldment, growth, and development as part of the spiritual path of humanity. It incorporates the creationist concept and the evolutionary process as the method of accomplishing this path.

Essential Oil Therapy interacts with other therapies in the most harmonious and effective way, incorporating techniques of both East and West. As people move through various stages the essential oils clear, cleanse, heal damaged auras, strengthen subtle bodies, and infuse light.

Essential Oil Therapy is not to be confused with aromatherapy, which is a more Western approach. The two are very different and come from very different understandings about how essential oils are applied, the responses they elicit, and the whole approach to the healing process.

Essential Oil Therapy addresses each individual as a universe. There is no set formula or oil that applies across the board. Each person is unique, and thus the expression of any one malady may come from different sources.

Therefore, the training given to therapists in classes does not focus on a standard way of using each essential oil. First, the therapist must focus on the individual and the internal processes of that person. One person may require a particular oil and the next person may have similar symptoms and require something entirely different because the underlying circumstances range widely. Ideally, each bath is customized for the perfect match. Since this is not a practical possibility, the formulas found in this book serve only as an introduction to Essential Oil Therapy. Even so, they should prove most beneficial. Therapists in all kinds of practices will find that training in Essential Oil Therapy will enhance and improve their practice in the most complementary way.

Essential Oil Therapy for children requires extensive and detailed instructions. It is a separate subject that is not addressed in this book, and should not be tried without supervision. Formulas in chapters six and seven may be used for adolescents fifteen years and up but may need to be cut to one-half or one-fourth strength for teens who are highly emotional, have been abused, or are involved in substance abuse.

1

Human Subtle Bodies

In the Western world we have identified so strongly with physical matter that we have come to believe that we are the physical body and that somehow our thoughts and feelings can be attributed to matter. Until we break the hold that this approach has on our attitudes and thinking we can never come to the reality and truth of existence. In my work with clients one of the most discouraging and frustrating situations I encounter is the difficulty in successfully communicating to them the concept of the existence of subtle bodies.

Grasping the importance of subtle bodies and integrating the concept as part of everyday awareness does not come easily to people; yet, it is critical to comprehending bath experiences and to overcoming the many fears that prevent us from moving forward. If the energy field is damaged, if there are gaping holes, if there is radiation, poisonous chemicals, or gases in the aura, then these things will make an impact on the vitality, strength, and overall health of the person. In fact, one can have a perfectly strong and healthy body, but if damage occurs in one or more of the energy sheaths, a gradual domino effect in the degeneration of one's health ensues.

Disabilities, weaknesses, food intolerances, emotional conditions, headaches, dizziness, menstrual-cycle problems, aches, pains, stiffness in the joints, sleep disorders, night terrors, depression, and, above all, confusion can be attributed to damage in the auric field. The list would run the gamut of human ills and even go beyond into areas not normally recognized or considered.

To my consternation and surprise, even students who have taken the training courses in Essential Oil Therapy often omit checking the condition of the aura of the client. The physical, emotional, and mental states are checked, but the actual condition of the bodies that are the emotions and mind are ignored.

Perhaps it is because the average person in the West is so stuck in materialism that trying to refocus the attention of the client into these subtle areas becomes too difficult and unrewarding. We seem to be so conditioned to healing by ingesting capsules, pills, and liquids that it becomes the path of least resistance. And so it is easier to gain the cooperation and understanding of clients by using familiar words and methods. Changing belief systems, entrenched habits, and attitudes is challenging and difficult. This is the reason why so much emphasis is put on energy, the subtle bodies, and the chakra system and the evolutionary process (as defined in the introduction) in these early chapters. For it is necessary to emphasize and, as forcefully as possible, to make the point that everything is energy. The physical level is transitory, a wink in time compared to the eternal light that we are.

Our greatest healing comes when we begin to investigate our subtle nature. For aside from accidents, contagious diseases, or exposure to radiation or other noxious substances, most of the physical ailments of humanity develop as a result of damage or negativity lodged in the emotional, mental, or soul bodies. Allopathic medicine treats the disease but misses the root cause of the disease, focusing solely on the physical level. The human energy field is largely ignored. Of course, once an imbalance has moved into the physical body from the subtle bodies, it is wise to use all means at hand to treat the problem. It is not a matter of doing one or the other.

Herbs are a wonderful adjunct to use with Essential Oil Therapy. They cleanse and strengthen the system. They kill infections and all sorts of invasive parasites and germs. They have been known to assist in strengthening the auric field, but it takes a very long time and sometimes much effort to find the right combination. The traditional herbalist works primarily with physical symptoms, acknowledging the mental and emotional condition. But herbs seem to work best on the physical level.

We stress this point because people frequently confuse herbs and essential oils as being somewhat comparable—and they're not. Both heal wonderfully, but they work in very different ways. While herbs are used primarily for physical symptoms, essential oils, as used in this therapy, have the power to cleanse and heal the aura in the most profound way. They neutralize irradiation in the energy field and heal holes, tears, and weak areas. They catalyze the clearing of negative pockets of emotional and mental debris, strengthening the energy field. They even pull past-life memories that may be strongly influencing the present

through the veil of forgetfulness into present consciousness so that people often are able to make a connection
with why they feel as they do toward certain persons or
situations. Getting in touch with these realities helps to
process and release old charged emotional pockets.

The dynamic properties of essential oils are such that
the instant a person enters the bath and sinks beneath the
water, healing of the damage in the energy sheaths begins. Let us now define and examine the seven human
bodies.

PHYSICAL BODY

There is little to say about the physical body that hasn't
already been said. Medical science has cataloged the physical matter and construction of the human body in great
detail. As electronics has become more important in the
practice of medicine, traditional medicine has begun to
recognize energy patterns within the human body. Eventually, as more information comes forth, science will likely
begin to seriously study the human energy field in a way
similar to the study of the atmosphere (or auric field) of
the earth. For there is a direct correspondence here. All
that we are is made of the elements that exist on the planet,
including our subtle bodies.

ETHERIC BODY

Each of the subtle bodies interpenetrates the physical body
and all other bodies it encompasses. The etheric body is
the blueprint for the physical body. We might compare it,

in some ways, to a three-dimensional circuit board. This is the body that provides the circuitry that receives energy from all the other bodies and conducts this energy into the physical body. More than that, it is the energetic pattern upon which the human form is fashioned. We have all seen the oriental drawings of the Buddha sitting in a lotus position in meditation. Lines run down his face and arms and over his entire body. These lines represent the energy currents that make up the etheric body. They are called meridians. The points where many of these meridians come together are called chakras. There are seven major chakras and twenty-five other chakras of secondary importance. The points where several meridians cross are called nadis, a Sanskrit word for which there is no comparable word in our language. These are considered minor chakras. They are tiny spinning wheels of light found at intervals over the entire body.

If the flow between the etheric body and the other bodies becomes clogged or the circuitry in the etheric body becomes jammed or disconnected, body systems and organs do not receive the vitalizing energy flows required, and a slow deterioration of the physical body begins. The deterioration may be almost imperceptible or it may be dramatic, depending on the degree and type of interference. Fatigue is one of the most common reactions. Symptoms such as listlessness, lack of stamina, or a constant need for sleep can be ascribed to a variety of causes but are often the result of aura damage. Eventually the condition leads to chronic problems, illness, and disease.

The etheric field extends approximately two to four inches beyond the physical body in the average person. In a person of great physical stamina the etheric field can extend as much as nine inches, but this is rare.

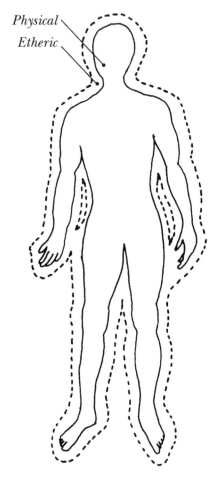

Physical
Etheric

TWO BODIES OR SHEATHS: PHYSICAL AND ETHERIC

The etheric body is more easily seen by the naked eye than any of the other subtle bodies. A simple exercise can train the eye to see it, using the following method.

In a slightly darkened room, seat a person against a white wall. Relax and unfocus your eyes. Do not look directly at the subject, but look a little to one side or slightly above the head. After a few tries a particular bright spot around the person may be noticed. Continuing to focus on seeing the energy field; it may come into your vision in glimpses at first. With practice it becomes easier. Usually the area around the crown of the head and across the shoulders is easiest to see. The quality, brightness, and width of people's etheric field will vary greatly. Once a person is proficient in seeing the etheric double, it becomes possible to see this energy field around fellow workers, family, friends, people on the street, or almost anyone, anytime, at will.

ASTRAL BODY

This body is the expression of the lower feeling nature. In teachings of the East it is called the body of desires. It is the body of attachment—attachment to all and anything that will gratify desire.

The astral plane is also called the watery plane. It is an unstable element that distorts the vision, just as looking through murky water distorts clear vision. It is the plane that swirls with mists. All of this applies as well to the astral body in humans.

Normally, when people with second sight speak of seeing colors around people or say they can see the aura, what they are seeing is the astral, or emotional, body. This body is more difficult to see with the naked eye than the colorless etheric body because it is made of a more refined substance.

We look out upon the world through our energy field. The condition and clarity of the etheric, emotional, and mental bodies color and affect how and what we see and hear. In other words, they affect the clarity of our sense perceptions and how we take in the situations and events around us. This is why eyewitness accounts of events can vary so widely. The power of observation is dependent on the ability of the person to be centered. The desired state is one of calm, clear, compassionate concern. The person who carries a weight of emotional and mental baggage will easily become polarized and emotionally involved in what is taking place, especially if the situation at hand is highly charged. Once this happens, everything becomes subjective, and objectivity flies out the window.

A person who has come into this life at an advanced spiritual stage and who has had a relatively normal and happy life will have an array of clear, beautiful colors swirling around him or her. It is also true that a person of spiritual stature may have an incredibly difficult life. The process of working through these obstacles produces much strength and insight. The colors in the aura of these people might be quite beautiful to behold. One might even see a great deal of white light, an indication of spiritual advancement of high degree. There is, of course, much more to the subject than is presented here.

We are the culmination of all that we have experienced and learned from our journeys through our many lives on this planet. People do not experience or learn in the same way or at the same rate even when put in the same circumstances. The person with clear and beautiful colors in the aura has, in this or other lifetimes, done much inner work of personal purification. We must all pass through the purifying fires of purging our inner demons in order to arrive at a point of clarity in our perceptions. There is one basic tenet to the attainment of elevated consciousness: purify, purify, purify.

Some time ago I attended a conference on radiation and breast cancer at the Lyndon B. Johnson Library at the University of Texas in Austin. One of the final speakers was Sissy Farenthold, a well-known political figure in the sixties and seventies who came close to being elected governor of Texas. She has remained a political activist behind the scenes, putting time and energy into areas of personal commitment.

As she stood at the lighted podium I suddenly became aware that I could see her aura. Ordinarily I don't see auras and don't look to see them. So I was both surprised and fascinated.

Her auric field was striking. Around the head was a soft, lovely, vibrant, clear pink. From the shoulders down she was enveloped in a cloud of beautiful powder blue.

Both of these colors are of a very refined nature. The pink indicates a highly evolved and selfless dedication and love for the planet. The blue is the reflection of one who is decentralized and who feels a love for humanity. This is the aura of a true world-server, always of value but especially so in these days.

The state of the auric field cannot be faked. Colors of beauty and clarity cannot be manifested at will. They are a reflection of the consciousness and level of spiritual attainment of the individual. For each of us, auric colors are indicators of the state of our spiritual progress.

In any given lifetime, when we die we carry with us the seeds of unresolved issues from that lifetime. These same issues will play out in lifetime after lifetime until we begin to understand how to deal with these issues and interrupt the repetitive cycle.

When I first began to work with essential oils I had a deep sense of mission and commitment to the therapy as it unfolded. I knew that it was sacred work and that the importance of the healing people would receive was beyond what I understood at that time.

For the first year or so, people came to my home through word of mouth from family or friends. Clients would take their baths, which I prepared and timed. After they had finished and dressed, we would sit together and talk about their impressions of the effects of the bath. Sometimes they were very present and were able to give clear descriptions of their experiences. Others seemed serene and abstracted, as though deeply internalized and processing.

The shift in demeanor, attitude, and facial expression of people before the bath and afterward is often dramatic to behold. The face becomes soft and relaxed. The mask we present to the world melts away and our true self is there, almost with the innocence of a baby. The skin is pink and rosy. There is a glow about the whole head that radiates as though one has been at the beach soaking in salt water and basking in the sun.

The emotional body seems to be the body that responds to the baths most quickly and easily. It is difficult to determine whether this is because most people are primarily emotionally polarized or because the essential oils simply affect the emotional body more strongly. Perhaps both are true.

For ten years I researched and documented the results of the baths. There are some astonishing stories. Aside from the expected results of stress release and improved sleep patterns, people began to relate that they were experiencing past lives. Often these were people who had never had a personal experience of this type, and some of them had no particular belief about reincarnation.

One woman in particular helped me understand the powerful healing process that can take place when we connect with these events from past lives that hold us in invisible bondage. This woman was a quiet, self-contained person, a massage therapist in her mid-to-late thirties. She spoke very little during the consultation, responding only when necessary. She came back for a second time, and when I asked her about her first bath she had very little to say. Her demeanor was flat, and I wondered to myself why she had come back because she seemed almost disinterested.

When she came back the third time I was quite curious but proceeded to put the formula together. Before I had finished she interrupted me by saying that she had something important to tell me. She then related the following:

As she was immersed in her bath she went back to the scene of her death in her last lifetime. She was lying in an open pit on top of a heap of bodies, looking up at a German soldier standing at the edge of the pit pointing a pistol at her. At the moment the soldier pulled the trigger, her dying thought on the horror of the atrocities she had experienced was *It is not possible that God exists.* For if God existed, these kinds of horrors would not be allowed. She died with this deeply despairing conviction.

As a result of reliving this event, the woman realized that she had carried the thought that God does not exist into this lifetime as her underlying belief. This was a stunning revelation for her because, although it *was* her belief, she had been completely unaware that this subconscious condition guided and controlled her entire life. In fact she stated that she was so surprised by it that personally reliving the experience was the only way she would ever have accepted this fact as a truth for her. She believed that no one would ever have been able to convince her that this was her deep conviction. Only because it was revealed to her in such a direct and personal way was she able to accept the truth of it and to look back over her life and see the reality of it.

Many of those who died in concentration camps during World War II have reincarnated and are dealing with a range of mental, emotional, and physical problems. I have had perhaps a half-dozen clients who have had past-life memories of being in concentration camps. From working with these few, I am convinced that this is the source of many cases of anorexia.

These are the kinds of dark clouds that we bring in with us from past lives for the purpose of clearing and releasing the negative charges and learning the life lessons that are there to be found. For the majority of people the purification and purging of these pockets of negativity in the emotional body are the primary healing steps to be taken. Understanding that these are steps to freedom and self-empowerment is important in releasing people from the fear of their own unworthiness or inability to deal with issues. This is a huge block for many people, and too often it seems to be the greatest obstacle to growth and progress.

It is a lie that we are unworthy. We are all beings of light, a part of and a reflection of the Godforce that flows through us. Fear, anxiety, insecurity, a sense of unworthiness, guilt, anger, and confusion obscure the light within.

One of the most important aspects of doing a bath series is that the act of being immersed and alone in a tub with an essential oil formula puts a person into a state that facilitates a connection with the inner self. As one sinks below the water and the cleansing of the aura begins, the focus turns inward. When this happens, the inner journey back to the soul begins. For the only pathway back to the light of the soul is the inner pathway. To face oneself alone can be to face one's innermost fears. This is an incredibly self-empowering act of courage. The power of the fear that keeps us frozen in place is that which we should be most concerned about and strive to overcome first and foremost.

MENTAL BODY

The mental body encompasses and extends beyond the astral body. The illustrations show the various egg-shaped bodies as approximately equidistant from each other. In truth, they pulsate and swirl, expand and contract, varying considerably in size in different individuals. In some the astral body may extend out from the physical body five or six feet while the mental body extends only a foot farther. In others the mental body may extend outward to seven or eight feet and the astral body may measure out to three feet. In the first case the state of the aura indicates that the person is emotionally polarized and may be carrying a heavy emotional weight. In the second case the indications are that the person is more mentally polarized and may be repressing the emotions. Occasionally it may mean that the person has processed and cleared at the emotional level and is well along with the integration of the three lower bodies.

In early evolutionary stages the focus was on the etheric-physical bodies. The integration and refinement of these vehicles was of paramount importance. As consciousness developed, the range and depth of the emotional nature came into play. The emotions held sway and reached a peak during Atlantean times. At a certain point in the development of the emotions in the human race, the

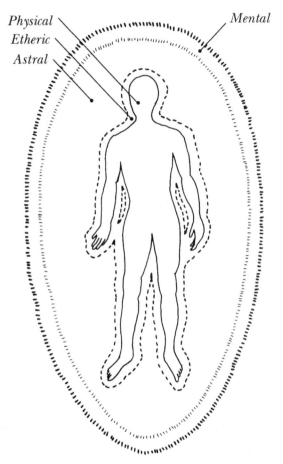

FOUR BODIES OR SHEATHS:
PHYSICAL, ETHERIC, ASTRAL, AND MENTAL

mental faculties began to be stimulated and the mental body in humanity took on a growing luster, strength, and clarity. This is a natural progression that is part of the evolutionary path of humanity. The development, refinement, and integration of these three vehicles—physical/etheric, emotional, and mental—is the immediate goal.

As we move outward from the physical body, each successive sheath is more powerful than the last and plays a role in integrating that which it encompasses. That which is greater encompasses that which is lesser. The mental body, or mind, plays a powerful role in bringing the emotional nature into a calmer state.

The emotional nature is a critical part of our makeup. In the earlier stages of development it is strongly influential in keeping us in an emotional state that is selfish and immature. Our feelings, when tempered and refined, bond us together and bring about harmonious relations. The integration of a refined emotional body and a developed and tempered mental body results in balance, intelligence, compassion, and an ability to express the true meaning of love.

These are three distinct vehicles, each of which must be as finely tuned as instruments so that an integrated balance can take place. This is necessary for preparation for the next giant leap for human evolution.

The mental body—literally the mind, the electronic energy field, which generates activity in the brain—is not as richly colored as the astral sheath. It is made of more subtle matter. As we think we manipulate mental matter unconsciously. Few people have the gift of sight that allows them to see mental matter. Those who can see in this way almost always either bring the gift with them from a past life or live in cloistered environments and undertake extensive training.

ENERGY FOLLOWS THOUGHT

As we conjure images in our minds of past events or present activities our thoughts form geometric configurations constructed of mental matter. These geometric

forms pop out of our heads and hover about until they
float away and dissolve. If they are highly emotionally
charged they have a longer life expectancy. Since strong
emotional charges are usually negative in nature—fear,
anger, lust, greed, etc.—they influence the immediate area
negatively. There are many people, mental types, who walk
around encased in thoughtforms. This is a major reason
why it is important not only to clear away negative emotional pockets but to monitor thoughts as well.

There was a remarkable woman who held a master's
degree in social work and conducted a private counseling
practice in Houston, Texas. After she had been practicing
for several years she developed a large following of ador-
ing clients. She often spoke to civic and church groups
and became quite well known in the Houston area. Her
name was Ann Barnett. We were lifelong friends from the
moment we met until her death.

Ann was gifted. She wasted no time on people who
did not want to get well, and she wasted no time in going
to the heart of the matter with clients. In fact, she told
me that if she couldn't break through and help clients
by the seventh session she did not feel that she could help
them. She was so good at what she did, so helpful with
her clients in loving and supporting them while guiding
them through their issues, that her clients were often
dazzled by her accuracy and ability to hone in on critical
issues. Many people who had been in therapy for years
would hear about her and come for help. It wasn't unusual for major breakthroughs to occur in the first or
second session.

Ann was brilliant, a genius with a heart to match. She
was also six feet tall—an imposing figure. Her hugs were
bear hugs. The love that she poured out to her clients was

returned to her in the great affection and tenderness with which people showered her.

One day I asked Ann how she was able to do this miraculous work. She told me that as she spoke with clients and they began to relate their problems, geometric forms would emerge out of their heads and hover about. She said that she could mentally engage these forms and, by doing so, experience what the clients had experienced. I asked her to describe to me what these geometric forms looked like. She said that there were many different kinds, but she looked for one in particular because she found it to be full of information pertinent to her counseling work. It was a little form that resembled a pig's tail with the end sticking up. She would mentally grab the end of the tail-like thoughtform and go into it. What she would see was an instant replay as though playing back a videotape. She was able to repeat conversations verbatim, even with the same intonations and emotional intensity.

I remembered having a book by Annie Besant in my personal library titled *Thoughtforms*. Annie Besant was one of the founding members of the Theosophical Society. She wrote several books, which are published by the

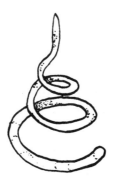

Thoughtform

Theosophical Press. *Thoughtforms* is filled with drawings
of these geometric configurations. Out of curiosity I
looked through the book to see whether there might be
something that looked like the form Ann had described.
Much to my delight, it is in the book.

The integration of the mind and the emotions takes place
when the mental energies begin to play on emotional matter. This happens not by suppressing the emotions but by
arriving at a certain maturity level. At this stage the person
senses that personal gratification is not the final answer to
things and begins to become less self-absorbed and more
interested in greater issues. Once this process starts and the
rays of the mind play on the clouded emotional body, spiritual advancement is hastened. The mind evaporates emotional mists much as the sun burns off mist in a valley. This
decentralization eventually leads to an expansion of awareness and a highly developed sense of responsibility.

A method that further hastens the process is to practice becoming the observer. This is a technique I encourage clients to use when clearing and releasing emotional
traumas in the baths or when there are fears or anger to
be dealt with. Once the emotions come up they should be
allowed to be felt. However, emotions cannot be cleared
and released if the fear or trauma takes over and the person is sucked under into an emotional whirlpool. This state
only results in a repetitive cycle. To break this cycle the
technique is to take a part of oneself during the bath, go
to the corner of the bathroom ceiling, and watch the emotions wash over oneself like waves. This is a neutral stance,
which neither feeds nor represses the emotional nature.
It is a process by which one learns self-understanding and
by so doing learns to understand others. When we stop
feeding the emotional storms by being willing participants,

these storms begin to atrophy. In this way we begin to develop wisdom and to find peace within. It is a process of emotional distillation, which eventually eliminates the gross qualities, leaving the more refined, cultivated qualities. The technique is a yogic spiritual practice and it works wonderfully. The baths make breakthroughs to emotional pockets that have been sealed away because of the pain, fear, shame, or whatever. "Out of sight, out of mind" is not a healthy state.

As the emotional, mental, and physical vehicles become more cohesive and made of a finer grade of material, the higher mind activates. This is the area in the mental sheath that extends from the outer edge of the emotional body to the inner edge of the soul body.

THE INTEGRATED PERSONALITY

At this point we will digress briefly from focusing on the subtle bodies and turn our attention to the components of the lower personality.

At the base of the spine in the etheric body is an energy coil of light. This energy material is coiled two and one-half times, and it rests quietly as if in slumber. In ancient tradition it is called the kundalini and often is referred to as the serpent.

When a fragment of the soul descends into human form it brings with it, encoded as DNA is encoded, characteristics, traits, abilities, and past-life talents and issues. All of what makes an individual unique is encoded in the kundalini. This coil influences who we are and how we express ourselves through the various sheaths in many lifetimes.

The combination of the kundalini, physical/etheric bodies (considered esoterically to be one body), and the emotional, mental, and soul bodies make up what has been termed the lower man or lower personality. This is a combination of five energies. The five-pointed star is a symbol that represents the five-fold nature of humanity during the lower evolutionary stages. Over our many lives we learn to wield energy through every conceivable combination of the five aspects that make up the lower personality.

As we incarnate over eons of time (esoteric and spiritual literature places the existence of humans on this planet long before history books do) we take part in the refinement of matter, influencing the quality and degree of light within matter through appropriating and raising the frequency of our sheaths and through influencing the atomic matter of the food and drink that we ingest. This is a constant, never-ending process because the ladder of spiritual evolution is continuous, stretching out before us into infinity. In spiritual terminology this process is called the *redemption of matter.*

As each vehicle is refined and as we incarnate over and over, we gain dexterity in our life skills. We develop and strengthen our perceptions and gain competence in working with matter. We deepen our understanding of self and others, and at some point we begin to attract and build into our vehicles matter of a finer gradation: matter that is more light filled. Through our personal effort we clear the murkiness and negativity out of our subtle bodies, and the light that we are begins to radiate and grow.

At a certain stage, when the lower personality begins to integrate, we attract the attention of those who watch on the inner planes. Our progress begins to be closely monitored. It is at this point, *for by our light they know us,* that those who aspire to a higher calling step onto what is called the probationary path. We are discussed, and the influence of these higher realms begins to be felt in our lives. As we sleep at night we are occasionally called into meetings on the inner planes and updated and encouraged on our progress.

The essential oils, as used in baths and massage, facilitate and accelerate this process in a way that is unmatched by any other therapy. The major reason is that the essential oils, sacred substances, heal the subtle sheaths in the most amazing way. The essential oils are able to put us in touch with our innermost being. They infuse light into all of our bodies. Getting into an essential oil bath is like getting into liquid light.

SOUL BODY

This is a body of light that shines brightly in the area between the higher mental body and the monad body. In the lower evolutionary stages, if we were to scan the outer areas of the soul body, moving into the dense body, we would find that the soul energy is all but obscured by the pollution in the mental, emotional, and etheric bodies. As this darkness is cleared the light of the soul begins to shine through.

The soul is present in the human being in four ways. It is present as a point of brilliant white light with a blue cast located in the center of the head between the pineal and pituitary glands. This point of light is attached to a silver cord made of the most beautiful and pure energy.

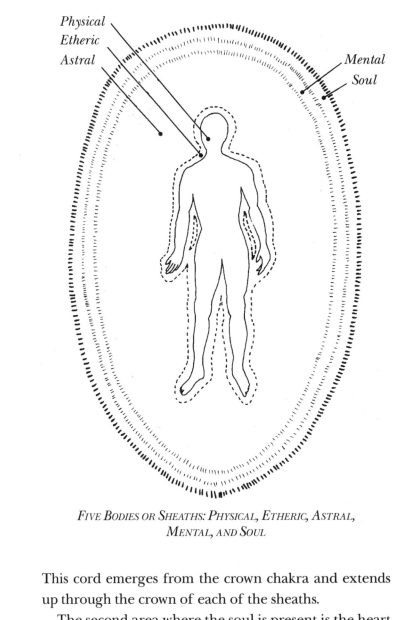

Physical
Etheric
Astral

Mental
Soul

FIVE BODIES OR SHEATHS: PHYSICAL, ETHERIC, ASTRAL,
MENTAL, AND SOUL

This cord emerges from the crown chakra and extends up through the crown of each of the sheaths.

The second area where the soul is present is the heart chakra. Soul energy pours into the heart chakra from the soul sheath. The soul is the expression of love and wisdom. The heart muscle is vitalized by a golden cord attached to the heart chakra. This cord comes from the crown point of the monad sheath and carries with it the life force that regulates the beat of the heart. The soul sheath, which encompasses and interpenetrates the mental, emotional, etheric, and physical bodies, is the third area. The soul is the higher source of our feeling nature. It's highest expression is love and wisdom. The soul is a part of our being, and the soul sheath begins to shine through and move into our awareness as we clear out lower vibrations.

Energy currents flow between the outer sheaths, into the etheric body, and from there into the physical form. Since the outer bodies are so difficult to see, not much is known about the energy flow between the sheaths. The condition and clarity of the sheaths govern the amount of energy that flows from the outer light bodies and into the chakra system.

There seems to be virtually no literature or information in the Western world on this topic. If there is more reliable knowledge in Eastern spiritual teachings I would suspect that it could be found in Tibetan teaching but perhaps taught only to those in training in the lamaseries. This is only a guess. Tibetan lamas are given very advanced training, and some of them are powerful healers.

The fourth presence of the soul in the physical/etheric vehicle is due to an activity known as the kundalini experience or the rising of the kundalini. At the culmination of this event the soul descends through the crown chakra and down the spinal column and seats itself where once the kundalini rested. After this takes place, the emotional or astral body begins to dissolve and is gradually absorbed into the soul body. This is the lifting up of the lower by the higher. It is perhaps what we could call a

heavenly marriage and is one of several initiation processes well recognized in the East.

Monad Body

The monad body is aligned with the Father aspect and is
an expression of will and power.

The energy of the monad does not begin to be felt
directly until after the kundalini experience. After further integration and purification, a greater infusion of
the monad occurs. At a certain point, the monad gradually absorbs the soul body in the same way that the soul
body absorbs the emotional body after the kundalini experience.

Logos Body

This is a body that represents planetary energy and to
some extent that of our solar system. Little is known about
this energy sheath. We probably are not, as yet, able to
interact multidimensionally at a level that would allow
much comprehension of this vehicle. That will come at a
later time.

Auric Damage

What are the causes of damage in the subtle body and
how does this damage occur?

We can be damaged at the very outset of life during the
birthing process. Long labor, medications administered,

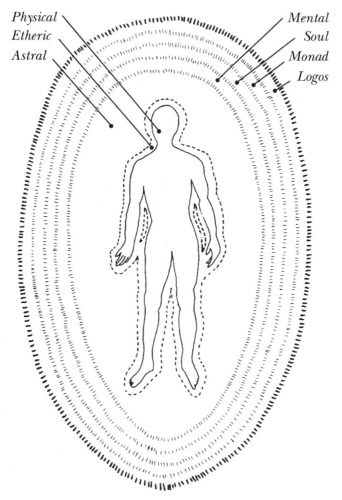

Physical
Etheric
Astral

Mental
Soul
Monad
Logos

SEVEN BODIES OR SHEATHS: PHYSICAL, ETHERIC, ASTRAL, MENTAL, SOUL, MONAD, AND LOGOS

complications in delivery, and difficulties in stabilizing after birth can cause damage.

Mothers who drink alcohol, do drugs, or even take medicinal drugs during pregnancy run the risk of blowing holes in the energy sheaths of their unborn children. It is a certainty that drugs and alcohol will do it. Medications may or may not, depending on many factors. Of course, this does not include the person who takes very small amounts of alcohol occasionally, though abstinence is best. Smoking can be a factor as well.

Damage in the auric field in infancy or while still in the womb can cause the most serious problems: lifelong problems that result in pain and disabilities for the child. For interruptions in the energy flow create flaws in the etheric body, which in turn translate to constriction of the normal energy flow. This especially affects the nervous system and the glandular system as well as the formation of the internal organs and the physical body in general.

Another source of complications caused by pregnancy problems is a loosening or partial detachment of the silver cord anchored in the crown chakra. This is a very serious injury because it is a partial disconnection from the soul. This condition may be one of the major causes of autism, mental retardation, and Tourette's syndrome. Experience in these areas has been limited, but because of the degree of success in these cases there is real reason to believe that healing can occur.

It is my personal conviction that auric damage is the underlying cause of attention deficit disorder and hyperactivity in children. Mothers who are at the end of their endurance have come to me for help. To date, each of these children immediately improved with the first bath. If the parents are committed and dedicated to staying on a disciplined bath schedule over several months, the child's behavior patterns become normal, provided there are no other circumstances that interfere.

A difficulty that I often encounter in treating children is that the parents do not follow through. Children rely on their parents to set the standards for their well-being. If there is stress, confusion, emotional upsets, or financial problems in the home, chances are that the child will not get the kind of guidance, focus, and attention required to follow a regulated bath regimen. If the child is older, strong-willed, or resistant, parents often haven't the staying power to insist and continue. Upon observing some of these families from without, situations can look hopeless in terms of the children getting the consistent help that they need. Even the most committed and well-meaning parents are all too often so immersed in their own life problems that they simply can't get it together to deal with anything more.

Barring other complications, once the damage has been repaired the nervous system seems to begin to function in a normal way. The child becomes more calm, able to focus, able to hear what is said, and able to respond appropriately. Temper tantrums and angry outbursts grow further apart. Nightmares, fear of the dark, fretful sleep patterns, and bed-wetting gradually diminish or cease completely. Appetite and eating habits improve.

The earlier this condition can be addressed, the better it is for the child and the entire family. Usually the child develops deep emotional scars over time. The out-of-control behavior creates a situation that makes the child a social outcast. Constant reprimands and recriminations lower self-esteem. Children know when something is terribly wrong and, as children do, they blame themselves.

It is not unusual in the initial bath series for a child to begin to cry with wrenching sobs during the second or third bath. When the mother asks what is wrong, if the child is old enough to understand and translate what is happening he often says that he doesn't know but that he feels so sad. This is the cue for the parent to wrap the child warmly in a towel and hold him closely, allowing him to cry as long as he needs to.

When children's antisocial behavior causes negative re-actions in others, this can be extremely painful and lonely for the children—isolation in a frightening world. They are often angry and always terribly frightened and confused.

The tearful outburst is a healthy release of these pent-up emotions. Essential oils erase negative emotions and heal the source of interference in such a way that the memory of the experience fades away and the person af-fected has to stop and focus deliberately to bring back the memories. Emotional scars and traumas are frequently completely erased.

It is my fondest hope that one day I will be able to ap-ply this therapy to infants and children born drug addicted or with fetal alcohol syndrome. I am convinced that many of these children could be greatly helped by Essential Oil Therapy. A well-rounded program is always desirable. In conjunction with using essential oils, I often recommend that people see other therapists for homeopathic remedies, special diets, herbs, and other such regimens.

Many children damage their energy fields from falls. Childhood diseases; chronic or serious illness; surgery; physical, emotional, mental, or sexual abuse; medications; being in or near an explosion; pollution; exposure to ra-diation; or ingestion of chemicals or heavy metals in the food chain can cause auric damage. In reality our chil-dren are seriously at risk in the present world.

If those who are responsible for the pollution only re-alized that their own families are at risk it might serve to turn things around. How can we expect children to even think straight, much less learn, considering the assault on their health that many endure? Baths, massage, and other methods of using essential oils are a simple and effective way to safeguard our children from some of these invisible modern menaces.

ENTITIES

The following discussion may seem strange and bizarre to readers used to a scientific interpretation of the universe, but for those unfortunates who have found their bodies weakened and their minds confused by entity attachment, recognition of the true nature of their problems has been a godsend to end a condition too long untreated. If the term *entities*, or the idea of beings that inhabit a realm other than the physical one, makes readers uncomfortable, please understand that these are concepts central to almost every religion on earth.

The term *entity* is used in spiritual terminology for many things. Because of the way it is loosely applied, the definition can be confusing. As it is used here the definition is specific. The atmosphere, or aura, of the earth has seven layers. The first is the etheric and the second is the astral, which interpenetrates the etheric and physical earth. This is a realm charged with human emotions, where strange apparitions can be seen. These apparitions are made of emotional matter, which reflects the state of emotions in the human and animal kingdoms.

The Catholic religion teaches of a place called purgatory, a place where the "wicked" go to remain until they have suffered sufficiently to redeem their "sins." This is the astral plane, the realm of spirits and ghosts.

Those who get trapped in the lower regions after death are those who die with unfinished business and are held back by their need for completion, people who are attached to their money and worldly goods, those who die under torture or long-term suffering and have become greatly weakened, those attached to family or loved ones in a codependent way, and, finally, those who have lived lives of extreme cruelty or depravity. If the personal frequencies of an individual have been so lowered, it becomes impossible to go into the light after passing over. It is impossible to see the light. These are the disembodied, which we identify as entities. They are discarnate humans who find themselves wandering about in a strange and unfamiliar place. They are lost and terrified. They exist in a neverending nightmare, trying to find a safe haven. They are somewhat like the homeless people of our plane. For the most part, these disembodied people are quite harmless, though they may have developed some bad habits, and many are undisciplined or have addictions. They seek out people to attach to so that they may reexperience human sensations, or sometimes primarily to escape the strangeness of astral realms and be in a more familiar and safe situation. Others who have addictions often seek out persons who have like addictions. Alcoholics and drug addicts with these types of entities attached to them have extreme difficulty because they are feeling the addiction of others.

In the modern world a new association with the astral realm has emerged. We have become a drug culture, not so much as a result of recreational drugs but more because our medical treatment has become primarily pharmaceutical. Drugs have become familiar and more acceptable as a result. Drugs damage the aura and lower the vibrational frequency of the energy field of humans. When the frequency is lowered, the light within the energy field is weakened and obscured.

People who live in nursing homes are regularly medicated. People who die in hospitals are often heavily medicated. Drug addicts and alcoholics who pass over have greatly lowered vibrational frequencies. Because of this, when these people make their transition they often cannot go into the light. Instead, they find themselves trapped in the lower regions of the inner dimensions, one of which is the astral plane. People who have damaged auras are wide open to these beings. Holes in the aura break the ring-pass-not seal that exists in a healthy energy field. Hands-on healers, who have the capacity to work with the energy field and heal damage, often seal the aura with their work. But this seal can be temporary and often ruptures again soon afterward. This is very similar to the functioning of the earth's atmosphere. In its normal state the atmosphere filters out and protects the earth from harmful rays from space. With the hole in the ozone layer we find that we are now being irradiated with a heavy dose of ultraviolet light. The ring-pass-not of the earth has been violated.

As Above, So Below

Once the energy field is damaged, the holes in the aura are like an open door for entities. Certain types of places attract these entities—places where people with damaged auras are likely to be found. They include bars, clubs, places where drugs are being used, recovery groups of different kinds such as AA meetings, hospitals, emergency rooms, nursing homes, scenes of disaster, battlefields, prisons, funeral homes, churches, mental wards, and homes for the mentally retarded.

This damage in the energy field does not necessarily heal of its own accord. Perhaps when we were more connected with the earth and out in nature, when our planet was not so polluted and the lifestyle was slower paced, we may have slowly healed in a natural way by swimming in clean lakes and streams or the salt water of our oceans, breathing in pure air and basking in the sun. Today this is not the case. We live in an atmosphere that has become so polluted that we are ingesting damaging elements in the food we eat and the water we drink.

When there are holes in the aura it leaves one vulnerable to parasitic entities invading the damaged bubble, much as bacteria invade an open wound. This damage leaves us vulnerable and weakened on many levels. Unless one has some kind of unusual spiritual dispensation and protection, when damage is present the person will almost always be host to entities, possibly thirty or more. This results in a drain on the nervous system and a depletion of the general energy level. Addictions of all kinds can develop, including sexual addiction. It even affects young children and is frequently responsible for premature sexual behavior.

As the person becomes weaker the desire and will of the entities gain more control, and the host becomes further confused and behaves in ways that are out of character. In some, this stage sets in after many years as the person grows older and weaker. With others, it begins in childhood or at birth.

Since essential oils heal the energy field in such a dynamic way, they also rout entities. The frequencies of essential oils are so high and light-filled that the entities cannot stay. The auric field begins to seal immediately upon entering an essential oil bath. The energy fields of the entities even receive some clearing and healing from exposure to the baths or to massage with an essential oil formula.

Each kingdom—mineral, plant, animal, and human—is on an evolutionary trajectory. Of these kingdoms, the plant kingdom has evolved on its own path beyond the other kingdoms. The spiritual criterion for evolutionary progress for each kingdom is the degree of planetary service rendered. This spiritual principle is a topic too vast to address here. However, to understand the power of the plant kingdom and its healing properties, it is necessary to touch upon the subject.

The plant kingdom has rendered and continues to render the greatest service to the planet above all other kingdoms. It provides the life support system for animals and humans. It beautifies the environment and brings solace and peace to the human heart. It stimulates joy, emits beautiful and healing fragrances, and provides shelter, food, clothing, and a vast array of artifacts such as paper and medicines. We could not exist for more than a few minutes without the oxygen that plants generate. Plants absorb and refine minerals so that they may be more easily digested and fully absorbed into the human and animal systems.

Each kingdom has a consciousness. Self-awareness increases with each successive kingdom, beginning with the mineral kingdom and moving through each to the human kingdom.

The essential oil is the most highly evolved element within the plant. It is the elevated nature of essential oils that makes them very potent healing agents. For if the human kingdom, on its own evolutionary path, were as advanced as the plant kingdom, we humans would be operating as conscious souls, and as a race we would be living lives that would bring love and wisdom to human affairs and thus to the planet.

Essential oils are the single most important element that provides people the means of accelerating their personal evolutionary progress. They are light-filled, and they evaporate darkness and negativity in the human physical, etheric, emotional, and mental bodies. They cleanse, allowing the soul to shine through.

Those who have auric damage should make careful preparations in advance of taking the first few baths in a series. Those preparations are as follows:

◇ First, call in your overlighting deva (guardian angel) and speak to it mentally, or verbally if you like, "as if" it is real and you can see it, even if you feel foolish in doing so. Tell it that you are aware of your situation, that you want to be healed and cleared, and that you request its participation and assistance in the process. Ask that the devas who receive and take those that pass over be present to help the entities go into the light.

◇ Acknowledge the entities and thank them for allowing you to serve them, as you have afforded them safe haven and even some possible healing.

◇ Tell them that you are going to begin the bath series and that you are going to begin to heal, so they may not stay attached to you any longer. Explain that they will get some of the same healing that you will get from the bath and that there is nothing to fear.

✧ Direct them to go into the light. Explain that there will be devas there to receive them and take them where they will be healed, safe, and happy.

✧ Then call in your own deva and ask that the devas who receive people when they pass over be present when you begin the bath. Ask that the personal deva of each entity, as well as relatives and friends on the other side, be present to receive each entity as it moves out of your auric field and into the light. Call upon help with this process from whatever spiritual realms or deities you are comfortable and familiar with. Do all this even if you are skeptical.

✧ As you get into the tub, ask that this process begin.

Before, during, or after the process, use any visualizations or phrases that seem natural to use. You may mentally or verbally talk with the entities and/or spiritual beings involved in the process. You may wish to meditate or pray for several days beforehand or afterward. There is no one way to deal with this, as the types of entities and the reasons for their being there vary greatly. Certain essential oils are specifically used for healing auric damage and for ejecting entities. Which of these oils to use is determined individually.

Some people have close relatives who have passed over who are attached to them. In these cases it is not always easy to let go. There may be a period of adjustment and grieving at the final "loss" of a loved one.

Sometimes there may be an entity attached that is unusually strong-willed and uncooperative, refusing to go into the light. As the baths are taken regularly, however, its hold on the aura will weaken and it must leave. Three or four baths may be needed to remove all of the entities, especially if they have been welcomed on a subconscious level and a codependent situation exists.

Essential oils are of the highest level of purity and refinement. They begin to heal damage in the auric field immediately. Entities benefit from the healing, but they cannot stay long within the auric field of one who is taking the baths, as the frequencies are too powerful.

People who have never had a psychic experience in their lives report actually seeing the entities and having mental conversations with them. Some say they "see" or "feel" them leave. Some experience the joy that occurs when the entities go into the light. Some sense the fear that the entities have. Sometimes there are very stubborn, resistant, angry entities who are determined to stay (to no avail).

If this process is not followed and the entities are not received into the light, they will be ejected out of the energy field and may hover about waiting for the chance to reenter their former "home," or they will wander off seeking another host.

2

The Chakra System
and Human Evolution

To understand the sensations and experiences that happen with essential oils, it is absolutely necessary to grasp the concepts and the consequent implications regarding the subtle bodies and the chakra system. The integration of this knowledge with what is known about the physical body provides us with a more complete understanding of who we are.

Contrary to many belief systems in the Western world, we are not static beings with one lifetime. We are eternal beings on an eternal journey, expressing our essence, expanding our experience, and learning about what creation truly is over many lifetimes. We are energy, manifesting as matter.

Through the appropriation of matter we imbue our light and our consciousness in minuscule portions to the atoms that compose our physical forms and to all matter that passes through our digestive system. Every atom is on an evolutionary trajectory.

43

The greater the clarity and purity of these seven sheaths, our subtle bodies, the greater the radiatory impact on matter.

As we progress on our journey we become increasingly radiatory. We expand our horizons, our understanding, our ability to become a part of the process of creation. We are, in fact, on the very same path as those great spiritual teachers, such as Buddha, Jesus, and Mohammed, who have gone before us and led the way. An understanding of the methods that propel us along our path provides us with insight into who and what we are, where we have been, and where we are headed. It presents us with myriad options that are part of the future, and it frees us of limitations. Our perspectives and perceptions change forever. By acting as a conduit that links the physical part of ourselves with the intangible parts, Essential Oil Therapy opens hearts and minds and clears the channels to spiritual realms.

However, all of this has little value if the understanding of what is taking place is misinterpreted, misconstrued, or experienced in a state of fear. Essential oil baths are not like any other experience. They are truly unique, as difficult to explain as a taste never experienced or a sensation never felt.

On our spiritual journey, the state of our chakras reflects the condition of our energy field. Each of the seven major chakras has a special relationship to certain glands and organs of the body and to one of the energy bodies. By monitoring our chakras we can maintain an awareness of the state of our subtle bodies. If there is a blockage in the subtle bodies due to damage, trauma, or unresolved emotional or mental conditions, it causes a block or shift in the energy flow to the chakras and thus to areas of the physical body. In every case to date, holes found in the auric field have been found in the chakras. These holes are blown out in a funnel shape similar to the chakra illustrations in this chapter. Sometimes these holes go through the etheric, astral, and mental bodies and extend as far as five or six feet, front and back. The illustrations shown are not true depictions of the chakras, which are said to look like partially opened blossoms that resemble the lotus. These spinning wheels of energy begin to take on colors of great beauty as we reach a certain point in our spiritual development. As the wheels pick up velocity the outer petals open and greater light shines forth, indicating progress in consciousness.

The seven major chakras are explored in this chapter.

CROWN CHAKRA

The pituitary gland is the master gland, which regulates the body systems. It in turn is regulated by the energy it receives from the crown chakra via the etheric body. The crown chakra is the most complex of the chakras, as all energies come together in a confluence at the crown. This chakra is called the thousand-petaled lotus. You will see it shown like a snug cap in drawings of the Buddha.

Examine the illustration of the crown chakra. Then examine the illustrations of the major and secondary chakras. Note that with the exception of the ear and eye chakras, all chakras pass directly through the body and have a magnetic and radiatory side. The front side of the body is magnetic. The back is radiatory. The crown chakra is the only chakra that is perpendicular and passes through the entire trunk of the body, emerging out the bottom of

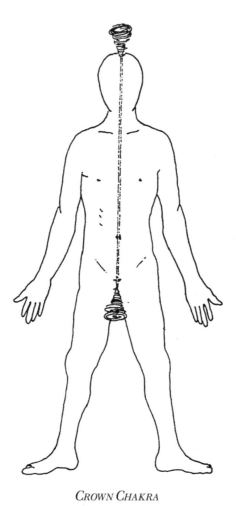

CROWN CHAKRA

the spine between the legs. This life force vitalizes the spinal column and all chakras along the spine, which sends this energy coursing through the entire body via the meridians. The crown chakra is radiatory and magnetic at both ends. The energies flow up and down the spine, entering and exiting simultaneously.

The true color of the crown chakra is red, the color that represents life, vitality, strength, will, and power. Red is a dominant color, and it has often been seen radiating around the root chakra. As this energy exits the end of the spine and mixes with colors of the lower chakras it can change to a murky, unappealing shade. The misconception of red being a color that is undesirable comes from this mixing of the energies in the lower chakras. None of the seven colors that combine to make white light are inferior to the others. They are emanations from Divine sources. The quality of the sheath matter through which these energies play determines the distortion or clarity of color. As these energies move through matter they strengthen what is there and are conditioned by the matter they move through.

Shine light through clear water and you get clear light. Shine light through murky water and you get distortion.

Energy is impersonal. It strengthens what is there. This is why it is so important to clear and heal before attempting to pull in more powerful energies through intent, focus, prayer, meditation, chakra stimulation, or any of the methods commonly used.

The fact that the chakras are said to be lotuses with petals that open seems to relate human circuitry to the plant kingdom. This is no accident, for there are always layers of meaning if we have the wit, will, and patience to follow them through.

In infants, the crown chakra is found at the soft spot on top of the head.

Ajna Chakra

Perhaps better known as the third eye, this brow chakra is the seat of intuition and telepathic abilities. It is the center

through which we interact with the devic or angelic kingdom. The ajna chakra is associated with the pineal gland—
something of a source of mystery, for the function of the
pineal gland is still not clearly defined or understood.

To find the location of the brow chakra, place a finger
on the center of the nose between the eyes. Run the finger
up the nose in a straight line until a small indentation in
the central brow area is felt. It will be found in slightly different locations on individuals but in the same general area.

The placement of the chakras has much to do with the
step-by-step unfoldment of humans and the built-in safety
features that prevent the overloading of our circuitry as we
progress. The soul is seated between the pineal and pituitary glands. This is the chakra that allows humanity to gain
dominion over the devic kingdom. That dominion is safe-
guarded in that one only gains access at such a time as one's
integrated soul/monad energies are in full control.

The true color of this chakra is green, though it is not
shown as green on any of the charts. Remember that we
are in a process of becoming. Colors that have been seen
playing through various chakras, with the exception of the
sacral chakra, have been shown to differ. The color seen in
a chakra may be for the purpose of balancing, vitalizing, or
harmonizing during a certain time period or stage. If the
true colors were to be flowing through fully opened chakras,
there would be only brilliant white light.

THROAT CHAKRA

This is the higher creative center. It is the higher octave
of the other creative center, the sacral chakra. The related
glands are the thyroid and the parathyroid, representing

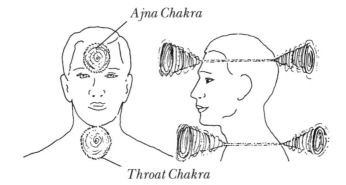

AJNA (BROW) CHAKRA AND THROAT CHAKRA

the uterus and ovaries in females and the testes and prostate in males.

When this chakra is fully opened and activated, the color yellow pours through it. The energy of this chakra in future will manifest as beauty and quality of speech in a way that is presently unknown. The meaning of the phrase "the power of the spoken word" will be better understood when this chakra comes into full expression. This is the chakra that represents the human race.

HEART CHAKRA

The heart chakra is a two-fold chakra. It represents the energy and center that is of utmost importance for the planet and all species upon the planet. It represents the critical step in the development of the human race. The lower center of the two-fold heart is the center of wisdom, and is the chakra directly over the organ itself. This center is vitalized and conditioned by the flow of soul energy through the chakra. The lower center opens first and directly stimulates the awakening of the higher heart chakra, located in the center of the breastbone between the thyroid and the heart.

In humanity there is a coupling of will/power and love/wisdom, as in the crown chakra, where we find the soul as a point of light in the center of the head, attached to the silver cord. In reverse we find the love/wisdom energy pouring through both chakras and the will/power anchored in the heart muscle by a golden cord. These two energies always work in tandem as balancing factors, playing out as the duality we find in each of us.

When we are born the thymus is very large in proportion to our bodies, and it is highly activated. The thymus is responsible for stimulating the immune system; consequently, infants in general have strong immune systems. As the infant grows into puberty the thymus gland becomes less and less active. It is as though we come into this world very connected to our life source, and as we become more deeply immersed in matter, forgetfulness sets in and that connection switches off.

As our spiritual journey continues, as each chakra is

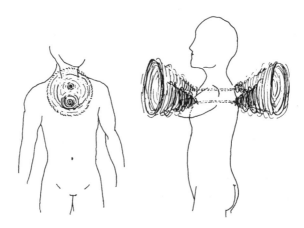

Two-Fold Heart Chakra

successively stimulated and the petals open, the heart chakra in adults will again stimulate the thymus gland into activity.

The gland related to the lower heart center is the spleen. The thymus is the gland for the higher heart center, sometimes spoken of as the will center.

The true color of this chakra is blue.

SOLAR PLEXUS CHAKRA

In various charts this chakra is placed in different locations by as much as six inches, and everywhere in between. Confusion abounds. This chakra is the seat of the lower emotions—anger, fear, guilt, jealousy, selfishness, and unhealthy desires. It is found directly beneath the sternum where the rib cage comes together, just over the stomach and only a few inches from the heart.

This chakra is the center most connected to the emotional body and the astral plane. The true color of this chakra is violet. The related gland is the pancreas.

The heart chakra is the higher octave of the solar plexus chakra.

SACRAL CHAKRA

Psychologists tell us that our sexual energy is represented by orange. This is the true color of the sacral chakra. On charts it is always shown to be orange, and it is the only chakra that always utilizes its true energy, radiating its true color. This is because it is the center of physical procreation, and as such it must be fed by the true energy.

In the womb, all fetuses begin as females. Chromosomes determine the gender of the fetus. During the very early stages of development, if the fetus is to be a boy, the uterus turns inside out as it descends and externalizes. The uterus becomes the scrotum and the ovaries become the testes. Because of this, the sacral chakra in females is directly over the reproductive organs, but in males it is about two inches lower and much nearer the root chakra.

In the illustration on page 54 the proximity of the exiting end of the crown chakra and the sacral and root chakras can be seen. The close placement of these three energies in the male body explains why males have such strong sex drives and why they are prone to be mentally and physically oriented. The will to be dominant is strong in this area of the body simply because these are the energies at play.

The solar plexus is located much further away from the lower three energies in males than in females. That

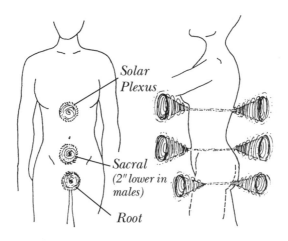

Solar Plexus Chakra, Sacral Chakra (Female), and Root Chakra

explains why it is harder for males to access their emotions. Males are polarized in the lower area of the spine because of the strong pull of the combination of energies in that region. It is much more difficult for men to access their emotional nature because of the pull of the lower region and the wide gap between the sacral center and the solar plexus center.

An awareness of this condition will greatly help men to understand themselves better. With this understanding they are provided the tools they can use to focus on the emotional integration required to move forward. The key for men is to work at finding the feminine parts of themselves and to consciously participate in the process of integration.

Many of the crimes committed by men are based on the mixing of the three energies in the lower part of the body. The only way that these energies can be refined and brought under control is through the integration of the feeling nature.

The energies of the sacral and root chakras are yang, or masculine, in nature, as is the opposite end of the crown chakra that exits between the legs. The combination of these three energies in such close proximity causes a strong and aggressive polarization in this region of the body that is devoid of the feminine (yin) feeling nature. Each of the chakras is of either yang, thought energy, or yin, feeling energy. When there is extreme polarization, as is present in the male body, it creates real barriers in balancing and integrating the thought/feeling energies. Integrating and coming to balance is the immediate evolutionary goal for the human race. It is the only way to open the heart.

The heart chakra, reached through the clearing and refinement of the emotional body and the solar plexus

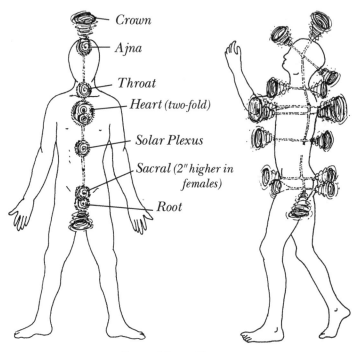

Crown

Ajna

Throat

Heart (two-fold)

Solar Plexus

Sacral (2" higher in females)

Root

SEVEN MAJOR CHAKRAS

center, is the key. Our lesson is to learn to open the heart and to give love. In so doing we serve. By serving, love is given in return. This is the only true way.

For men this is the most difficult hurdle, even when they are aware and willing to make a true effort. A case in point is that of a young man who recently came to see me for a consultation. This young man reflected a type of male that has become more and more common. Intelligent, informed, and dedicated to his personal growth, he had done a great deal of searching and studying. At the time he came to see me he had just finished a complete Rolfing series and was midway through a series of rebirthing sessions. The therapist for his rebirthing sessions had been trying to get him to release some blocks by crying, but try as he might he had been unable to do so. Through word of mouth he heard about Essential Oil Therapy and decided to have a consultation and get a personalized formula for a bath series.

When he came for his session we talked about the essential oils called for in his formula. They addressed the same issues being brought up in his rebirthing sessions and were very specific, going back to some traumatic childhood events.

He took his written formula; collected the essential oils, cider vinegar, and stone; and began his bath series. About three weeks later he called to say that there had been a major breakthrough. He recounted the experiences and subtle changes that took place in the first two baths. Then he took the third bath on a Friday evening. The next day his emotions began to come up and he started to cry. Once he had started, it was as if a dam broke. He couldn't stop. He cried all day Saturday and all through the next day. When he finally stopped he said he felt great relief, as if a huge weight had dropped from his shoulders. He felt lighter than he could ever remember.

It is quite an amazing revelation for a person to reexperience the pain and wealth of feeling that has been repressed over years of time. How we can carry this much without having a clue that it is there is a marvel; yet, it is quite a common situation.

The sacral chakra has powerful energy coursing through it, which can play a siren song. In its lower expression it is the energy of thralldom. It can be used to deceive and to hook us with the promise of pleasure. This is the chakra through which dark energy may be injected into our auric field.

If people only realized the chances taken with promiscuous sex (beyond the chance of physical disease), far more caution and consideration would be given to the selection of sexual partners. Blind lust, careless sexual gratification, sex and drugs, sex and alcohol are dangers to the soul. They can lead to entrapment by the dark side which can take many lifetimes to wrench free of and to be healed. This is why sexual acts are routinely used in cult rituals.

The line between healthy sex and unhealthy sex is clearly drawn. Where there is integrity, a sense of responsibility, and an honoring of the partner, the intent is appropriate. Where there is love between the partners, there is a balance of the thought and emotional energies. The balance of these two energies acts as a safeguard.

The sacral chakra represents the formation of energy into matter. The glands of the sacral chakra are the ovaries in females, the testes and the prostate in males.

Root Chakra

This chakra is located at the tip of the spine in the back of the body and at the pubic bone in front. It is the chakra that is most closely aligned with the physical body and is the energy vehicle that feeds and vitalizes the physical body.

Often this chakra is blown out in women during childbirth. Once the damage is done it can last a lifetime, and it causes a tremendous depletion of vitality. Left unhealed, it stresses the nervous system and can be the source of many physical problems. If the sacral chakra is also damaged it can cause menstrual-cycle trouble, miscarriages, or difficulty with conception.

Children very often damage this chakra in serious falls. Given the natural vitality of children, the damage in the aura sometimes does not manifest itself until the child moves into prepuberty or puberty.

In her book *Wheels of Light,* Rosalyn Bruyere, a noted healer and psychic residing in southern California, states that when she observes the root chakra, she can see a band of indigo light. The root chakra is closely linked vibrationally with the crown chakra; it is the lower octave of the crown.

The true color of the root chakra is indigo.

The glands are the adrenals, the fight-or-flight glands, which galvanize the physical body into action.

HEAD CHAKRAS

Aside from the two major centers—the crown and ajna chakras—there are five other head centers of significance. They are

- ✧ The tip of the nose. The opposite end of this chakra is the indentation at the base of the skull. This is known as the medulla chakra.
- ✧ The indentations at the temples.
- ✧ The jaw joints below the ears.

The head is a terminal where all the body's circuitry comes together. All of the head chakras radiate directly into the core of the head in the region of the pineal and pituitary glands.

The ear chakras combine the energies of the sacral and solar plexus chakras. The lower part of the face correlates to the lower trunk of the body. The eye chakras combine the energies of the heart and throat chakras, correlating to the upper part of the trunk of the body. The base of the skull correlates to the root chakra, both having to do with systems of the physical body.

Lung, Spleen, and Hara Chakras

In order of importance after the seven major chakras are the five head centers plus the two lung chakras, the spleen, and the hara.

The lung chakras are located between the thymus and the heart at each side of the breastbone. They are a bit difficult to find. Run the finger down the edge of the breastbone to a point where there is an indentation at each side of the breastbone. The lung chakras are about midway between the thymus and the heart. In the back, they are the point of tension between the upper part of the shoulder blades.

These chakras are often blown out when there has been child abuse, battering, or sexual abuse. Damage in these chakras can be the underlying cause of all sorts of lung disorders, including collapse of the lung.

The lungs are, of course, an expression of our life force. Breath is the signature of life. Lungs are the primary organs that retain the emotions of grief and sorrow. Karmic situations that get restimulated are some of the most difficult lung problems to clear. Past-life rape and strangulation has come up with clients more than a few times.

The spleen chakra is located on the left side of the rib cage just below and slightly under the last rib and near the lower left side of the stomach. It acts as a conduit for

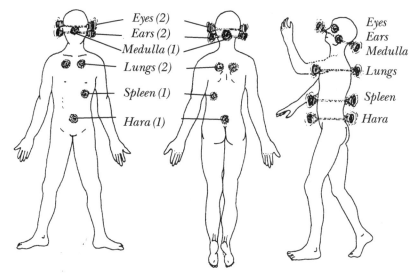

Eyes (2)
Ears (2)
Medulla (1)
Lungs (2)
Spleen (1)
Hara (1)

Eyes
Ears
Medulla
Lungs
Spleen
Hara

SECONDARY CHAKRAS (NINE MOST IMPORTANT)

the energies that flow between the sacral and throat chakras, rerouting it around the heart. Until the sexual energies have been refined and the solar plexus chakra has opened fully, the coarser sexual energies must be rerouted to prevent damage to the heart.

The hara chakra is immediately below the navel. It is often mistaken for the solar plexus. The hara is a center that was developed and utilized in the early stages of human development. It is the center of gravity and is the chakra that is focused upon in martial arts. I have seen yogis trained in utilizing this chakra who have defied groups of young men to lift them. Despite all efforts they cannot be budged. It is called a will center, and in a sense it is, as it is the center for the umbilical cord and thus a center of life force. It is also the center by which we carry with us our mother connection. It is the center through which many issues surface, as people are often connected to their mothers by an ethereal umbilical cord, which can be parasitic on either end.

Responses to the baths often mirror deeper tensions in individuals if one understands the signs and how to interpret them. The following case is one such example.

A young man living in the eastern part of the United States had requested a bath formula from me. A year after his formula had been sent to him, he telephoned one evening. He had waited for a full year after collecting his essential oils and other ingredients to take his baths. That night he had just taken his first bath. He said that he had just gotten out of the tub and there was a rash on his stomach. I asked him precisely where the rash was—up high under the ribs, around the mid-section, near the navel, or below the navel?

He said that there was a band of red rash that went completely around his body centered almost exactly over the navel.

I asked him how his relationship with his mother was, and for a few seconds there was dead silence. In a very quiet voice he said that this was the issue he had been working on.

Rashes and all forms of skin irritations are expressions of pent-up anger. When they come up in the baths, and they frequently do, they dissipate and vanish as the anger leaves. The skin condition is simply an indication of the amount and degree of anger. The area in which the skin manifests blotches or rashes indicates where the anger is lodged. Thus, an understanding of chakra energies and the organs associated with each provides clear clues to the kind of anger and the source of the problem.

The final sixteen chakras as shown in the illustration pinpoint the exact location of the chakras for the joints. For

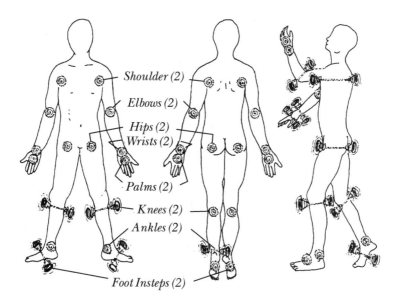

Shoulder (2)

Elbows (2)

Hips (2)
Wrists (2)

Palms (2)

Knees (2)

Ankles (2)

Foot Insteps (2)

SECONDARY CHAKRAS (FINAL SIXTEEN)

present purposes there is no need to go into further detail except to say that these areas often hold lodged anger, which manifests as joint stiffness, rheumatism, or arthritis.

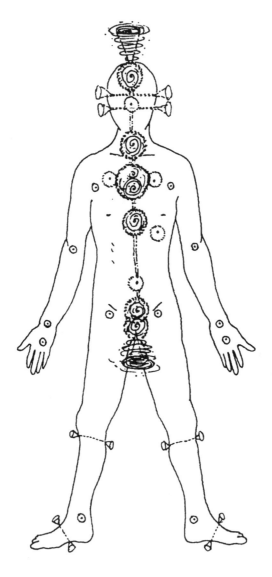

CHAKRAS: SEVEN MAJOR CHAKRAS,
SECONDARY CHAKRAS (NINE MOST IMPORTANT),
SECONDARY CHAKRAS (FINAL SIXTEEN)

3

Essential Oils and Their Healing Properties

The use of essential oils dates back to earliest recorded history, but in the past, essential oils were not readily available to the populace. Until modern technology was developed, the growing, harvesting, and extracting processes were so laborious that only the privileged elite had easy access to them.

Essential oils are extracted from all parts of plants and trees: flowers, leaves, bark, stems, resin, peels, rhizomes, and roots. The part of the plant or tree from which an essential oil is extracted will vary by species. For instance, essential oil extracted from violet leaves is different in quality and cost from that extracted from the petals of the violet flower; yet, both are quite useful.

Essential oils are the most powerful healing substances within the plant kingdom. Essential oils are extremely concentrated and potent; fifty pounds or more of plant matter is required to extract half an ounce of oil. For the

precious oils made from the petals of flowers such as orange blossoms, jasmine, and rose, hundreds of pounds of
petals are required to extract very small amounts. This is
why precious oils are so expensive.

There are several means of extracting essential oils. Steam
distillation is perhaps the most common means. Citrus peels
are cold pressed. Essential oils called absolutes are processed
with alcohol and solvents to extract the oils. This is the
method used for precious oils and for resins.

Essential oils are diverse in color and consistency. Some
are clear and colorless, while others are shades of yellow,
gold, brown, orange, and blue. They may be very thin and
runny, almost watery, or they can be as thick as molasses,
with a wide range in between. When essential oils are
mixed for a bath and poured into the bath water, they will
float at different levels, according to their consistency.

Vegetable and fruit oils are not to be confused with essential oils. Vegetable oils are extracted primarily from
nuts, seeds, and grains. They are thicker and more fatty
than essential oils. When placed in a tub with water, they
will float on the surface of the water. The molecules of
these oils do not penetrate the skin.

A minute amount of essential oil does penetrate the
skin during the bath, producing a deep heat that feels like
tiny suns moving through the bloodstream. The oils penetrate so deeply that the heat can be felt down to the bone
marrow. This heat can confuse the senses, and clients have
occasionally claimed that their bath water stayed hot for
forty minutes or more when we know that after fifteen or
twenty minutes the bath water cools substantially. Essential oils are volatile—they evaporate quickly when exposed
to air. This is an important point to remember. When they
are poured into a tub of warm water, the heat of the water

further hastens the evaporative process. Do not pour the oils into the water until you are ready to step into the tub.

During an essential oil bath, the cleansing properties of the oils work on clearing the auric field. They enter the physical body as they are breathed into the lungs.

Most people have not yet been exposed to a wide variety of essential oils. Rosemary, patchouli, lavender, and tea tree are probably the oils with which people are most familiar. Including the precious oils, there are approximately one hundred and twenty essential oils available, though no one company has all of them.

The healing properties of essential oils run the gamut of human ills and difficulties. I have yet to find a situation for which essential oils don't help in one aspect or another. For instance, the oils can't do anything about a broken bone; the bone must be set. But a medical person trained in Essential Oil Therapy could use the appropriate oils to reduce swelling and trauma and to keep the patient grounded and present.

One of the most critical problems in emergency rooms is keeping patients conscious and alert so that information may be gathered as they are being treated and examined. Camphor is the oil to use to keep people grounded and present—even to revive them. Eucalyptus is also grounding and clears the senses. Lavender might be called on to soothe and calm the patient.

Certain essential oils reduce swelling and dissolve the discoloration of bruises. They are so fast-acting in this regard that a sprained ankle can shrink back to nearly normal almost before the eyes, as though one were watching a film that has been speeded up. I have seen large, dark purple bruises completely vanish overnight after having essential oils applied.

Using essential oils in an environment where there are groups of people working together, such as a hospital or emergency room, can be very tricky because most people have issues they have not dealt with, and the essential oils can play on all these dynamics simultaneously. Problems of a most surprising nature can occur. This business of clearing out emotional baggage is tricky.

One of my earliest clients who now uses the essential oils in her thriving practice related an experience she had in her office. An acupuncturist shared the office with her. Between them they had many people coming in and out of the office each day.

One day she had occasion to use one drop of onion essential oil on a client. This one drop permeated the entire office, spreading to the reception area and moving beyond closed doors into every nook and cranny. The smell stayed in the office for two entire weeks. It was an experience that was hard to bear for all involved.

More than one student has related to me the uncanny way the oils have of traveling from one end of a house to the other to reach a person who needs them or to clear away negativity in an area.

Onion and garlic are the two most powerful cleansers in the spectrum of essential oils. Onion specifically addresses rage, anger, resentment, and other charged issues concerning male authority figures. Apparently a lot of masculine rage had been building in the office and needed to be cleared. It took a much longer time for one drop to clear it than if the appropriate number of drops had been used. When the negativity and the issues are cleared out, the smells do not linger in this way. This is a fascinating phenomenon of essential oils.

Essential oils are the original antiseptics. Many of them have one or more of the following properties: antibacterial, antiviral, antidepressant, antifungal, antiseptic, antispasmodic, diuretic, decongestant, astringent, antivenin, and many others. I once was called upon to use the antivenin properties of Essential Oil Therapy.

One day I stopped to see my son at his home. He had just returned from the doctor's office with prescriptions for antibiotics and analgesics. He had been bitten on the inside of the left forearm midway between the wrist and the elbow by a brown recluse spider. Several hours had passed since he had been bitten. The area around the bite was swelling and looked seared and red. A bright red streak stretched from the bite to his wrist, and in the other direction it almost reached his armpit. My son was beginning to feel nauseous, and the arm was beginning to throb with pain.

I asked him why he was given prescriptions for antibiotics and pain pills and was told that there was nothing to counteract the poison. The antibiotics were to prevent infection, and the pain pills were to numb the pain as the poison began to move through the bloodstream, affecting his whole body.

The red streak had moved up to the armpit and was continuing to move toward the heart. I became very alarmed. Brown recluse spider bites are very serious. I have been told that they act similarly to rattlesnake bites, but I had never seen or worked with either.

The spider's venom rots the flesh around the bite. The flesh turns black, and a chunk of flesh, like a plug, falls out. Unlike a rattlesnake bite, the bite of a brown recluse spider usually is not felt, making it difficult to identify the source of the problem until the body begins to react.

Normally people are bedridden and very ill for days after being bitten by a brown recluse spider. Some people become very, very ill. A few have even died.

Fortunately I had my essential oils with me. I collected them and brought them into the house. Having had such wonderful and helpful experiences with the oils, I felt certain that they would, in some way, be beneficial. My son sat down at the table with me. Using kinesiology, I checked him for the oils needed for the wound.

The essential oils called for were citronella, Peru balsam, and cinnamon. Citronella is one of the oils used to repel insects. In the definitions for the oils that I have received from the overlighting deva of each oil, citronella transmutes gloom into joy. It is an oil that exudes lightness and a sense of joyousness. Peru balsam neutralizes the residues of abuse. Cinnamon neutralizes anger. It is the master oil for anger.

In terms of understanding the energy exchange between the spider and the cells affected in the arm, the bite projected the energy of *anger,* a *suppression of life force,* and the *intent to wound.* The oils that were called for were more potent than the poison, overriding the negative energies with their positive ones.

I rubbed a mixture of these oils on the bite and from the wrist to the armpit, following the red streak. I soaked a large cotton pad with the three essential oils and placed it over the bite, binding it with gauze and tape.

My son was feeling sick and went to bed. An hour and a half later he awoke and came into the living room, where I had been waiting to check him.

When I removed the cotton pad and looked at his arm, all I could see was a small red mark where he had been bitten and some swelling around the bite area. The red streaks were completely gone. The swelling had gone down, and most of the redness around the bite area was gone. In addition, my son felt fine and the arm no longer throbbed.

I wrote out directions for him to soak his arm thirty minutes each day in a small tub of water with a mixture of the three essential oils and raw, unprocessed apple cider vinegar. He was to keep the bite covered by the cotton pad with essential oils on it.

He was able to go to work and suffered no ill effects from the bite except that after several days it formed a boil-like sore with a head. As it filled with pus it became heavier and more painful. At the end of the week it burst and drained. That was the end of it, and today there is not even a small scar to indicate where the bite was.

Essential oils are also used in surgery. Because of the antiseptic qualities of benzoin absolute, a resin, it is painted on the chest or abdomen or wherever the incision is made to sterilize the area. As it dries it makes the skin taut for a clean incision and closure process.

The essential oil of the plant is the true signature of the plant. The fragrances are sometimes surprising. Celery seed, for instance, does smell faintly like celery but has a much more biting, almost peppery smell. Black pepper essential oil has no bite or hot quality at all. In fact, it has a soft, sweet fragrance. The smell of lime essential oil is nothing short of exquisite.

A trained essential oil therapist can mix a personalized formula for a client that is as tailored to the individual as a designer garment. The formula should address the issues and needs that are activated at that time. These are very effective formulas because they are fine-tuned to the person's specific energy field.

Usually clients receive a written formula for a series of baths. The client purchases the essential oils indicated and takes a series of baths at specified intervals, following written instructions. Since each bath clears and shifts the energy field to varying degrees, the bath experiences and sensations can vary widely with each successive bath even though the same formula is being used.

The physical body responds in unusual ways to essential oil baths. Events that have been traumatizing leave energy tracks in the subtle bodies. During the bath, as the residues of these events are loosened and begin to disintegrate, specific configurations often appear on the skin. These configurations may be geometric forms, a handprint, belt or strap marks where one has been beaten, even marks like sores where one may have had some severe infection. The way the oils interact with the human body is parallel to the way developing solution works on film. The oils bring that which is invisible and unremembered to the surface, not only loosening the energy so that it can be released but giving tangible evidence of what we carry unseen and unfelt within us.

These skin markings can vanish as soon as one steps out of the bath, or it may take hours, days, or weeks, depending on the severity of the trauma and the ability to release it.

A case in point is a client who was on a very dedicated path of growth and service. She has spent much of her time in pursuit of personal growth, investigating various healing modalities and searching for spiritual truths. She is a spiritual warrior, prominent in her community, running her businesses with intelligence, and active in community affairs. She lives in a beautiful home, graciously appointed, and she routinely makes her home available for various meetings and spiritual groups, acting as facilitator and hostess. This woman, who is quite beautiful and still young, seems to have all that anyone could ask for.

After she had done several bath series, I began to have a nagging sense that she was still controlled by something very deep that had not surfaced. An underlying fear was present on a subtle level, and she was continually agitated and on guard even though there was nothing in her present life to cause this fear.

When I spoke to her about what I was sensing, she agreed that something was there but she did not know what. As we talked she had some sense that it was from a past life. We both felt that it might have been a sexual assault.

Because she is a most courageous and strong-willed person, and because the baths were not releasing the trauma, I suggested to her that a formula for a douche might do the trick. We spoke at length about how this might be accomplished, and once a procedure was decided I wrote out the formula. She was to do five douches at specific intervals.

A week or so later I received a phone call from her. She had just done the second douche and was standing in her bathroom in front of the mirror looking at a large darkly bruised handprint on her throat—clearly a man's large hand.

Our supposition had been correct. She was carrying the rage and terror of being raped and strangled in a past life. She had called for the essential oils that address anger and rape issues in all of her baths. No violence of this degree had ever happened to her in this lifetime.

After her phone call I did not hear from her again for some time. Later, when we spoke over the phone, she was deeply involved in community affairs. The underlying sense of tentativeness was gone, and she did not speak of the bath experience. She seemed to have dropped the fear, as though shedding a garment, and erased it from her life. She was busy, self-assured, and focused on her present life. This often happens with clients, for when the source of interference in their lives is removed, they seem to get a stronger direction and become very involved in following that direction.

The way that essential oils release negativity is most curious to observe. It isn't just that we assimilate an understanding, or forgive ourselves and others. The oils have an erasure action that completely removes these energy charges to the degree that the event seems never to have happened. Often I have commented to clients who have cleared highly charged emotions only to have them look at me blankly as though they didn't know what I was talking about. Sometimes I need to go over stories they have related to me in detail in order to jog their memories. They are so freed of the emotions that they need to reach for the memory as if it had happened to someone else long ago.

Again, a caution must be added. Essential oils are very potent. Unless one is a trained and experienced therapist, one should never attempt to put together a formula for a douche. Many elements must be considered before such action may be taken. The above situation is one of two times, to date, I have written a formula of this kind. The story is related for the purpose of underscoring the highly personal and individualized ways in which Essential Oil Therapy may be applied and the dynamic and often surprising results that the therapy brings about.

Regardless of the type of experience each person has in the baths, there are common threads that seem to run through the bath experiences with everyone who remains on a committed long-term program.

The first commonality is that the process of being in the bath alone and under the water has a stilling and calming effect that starts an internalizing process. For many people this is a new and moving experience. For the first time a process of looking within is begun. People begin to probe their own depths. This is the process that leads to discovery of the light within and that eventually leads to connection with our own higher soul-selves. This soul energy begins to guide us through life with a clarity and a knowing never before experienced.

It is impurity imbued in our bodies and our energy fields that prevents the light of the soul from shining through in each person. Healing the auric field, cleansing the emotions, and ejecting negativity from thought patterns are the keys to building a vehicle that is suitable to house soul energy.

Time and again, clients report a subtle and important shift in their perceptions and ability to see patterns in their lives after undergoing a series of baths. Problem solving is one of the most commonly reported experiences—the ability to see the subterranean energies that direct and govern our lives. This is incredibly self-empowering.

4

~~~~~~

Apple Cider Vinegar
and Gemstones
in the Bath

Apple cider vinegar has been praised for its healthful and curative properties for centuries. In Europe, especially in Germany, apple cider vinegar baths are still a regular part of a preventive health regimen. Numerous books in the United States expound the health properties of apple cider vinegar. From the first bath I ever prepared, which was mixed for a family member in extreme stress, apple cider vinegar has been an ingredient in my formulas.

The therapy that has evolved did not come from a consciously formed intent. Whatever name it might be called—inspiration, intuition, revelation, etc.—the combination of ingredients came to me in a flash of knowing. That first bath had apple cider vinegar, a clear quartz stone, and a combination of essential oils. These three ingredients have been part of the basic foundation upon which Essential Oil Therapy rests. Every formula calls for natural, unprocessed apple cider vinegar and a particular stone.

Apple cider vinegar is said to nourish the tissues of the skin and to open the pores. The most probable explanation for the benefits of vinegar in the bath is that the acidic property of the vinegar breaks up the droplets of essential oils so that they mix better with the bath water. Apple cider vinegar in the bath also solubilizes minerals, softening the water. In addition, it restores the pH balance of the skin.

Natural apple cider vinegar contains malic acid, an ingredient that cleanses the body of toxins. It also contains potassium, phosphorus, natural sodium, magnesium, natural fluoride, iron, silicon, sulfur, and many other trace minerals.

The natural vinegar is dark and has cobweb-like streaks through it, called the mother. The best apple cider vinegar is grown organically and aged naturally in wooden casks. Commercial apple cider vinegar is distilled. The vinegar is heated and turned to steam. The distillation process kills the enzymes and removes the mineral content. Commercially produced vinegar, devoid of minerals, makes a very weak electrolyte solution. The natural vinegar's mineral content allows it to conduct electricity more easily.

All matter, even atoms, has an etheric double. Living things have an etheric double and an astral field around them that produces colors. This gives their etheric fields an infusion of life force, which is imparted into matter. The crucial difference between the major brand-name companies who sell vinegar through the supermarkets and the whole vinegar sold in health food stores is the degree of life force retained in the vinegar when the vital elements are not removed.

The combination of essential oils, natural apple cider vinegar, and a quartz crystal or other stone makes a mixture that amplifies the healing properties of all three. Removal of any one of these ingredients changes the impact on the energy field. The water, vinegar, stone, and essential oils combine to make a healing soup for the human energy field.

A clear quartz crystal is used in many of the bath formulas in this book. It is used because it is adaptable, not because it is the best or most accurate energy for each individual. In private consultations people almost always call for a particular stone or combination of stones. Clear quartz crystals are seldom the stone used.

The stones my clients most commonly call for are amethyst, azurite, citrine, emerald, purple fluorite, garnet, jade, lapis, malachite, black obsidian, peridot, clear quartz, rose quartz, ruby, blue sapphire, sugilite, topaz, and tourmaline (all colors).

Of the stones listed above, the stone most often called for in formulas is lapis. About eighty percent of the personal bath formulas have a lapis stone in them. In descending order, the other stones most often used are black obsidian, sodalite, and rose quartz. Other stones are used occasionally. Diamond is not listed because to date only one client has used a diamond in a bath series.

Stones that are cut and polished can be used if they are the only ones available. It is better than having no stone. The preferred stones are not shiny, polished ones, but those in their natural state, preferably with some of the matrix (the portion of the rock to which the stone is attached) still intact. A natural stone has more life force and performs better in the bath water.

One should take great care when substituting stones for those listed in the formulas. This can backfire and cause temporary distress. Clients have reported experiences they have had as a result of leaving the stone out, either on purpose or by accident. When they got into the water, suddenly their bodies felt as if they had caught on fire. They immediately got out of the tub and the burning subsided. Placing the stone in the water, they reentered the tub and found that they could sink down under the water with no unpleasant reaction. Of course there must have been clients who failed to put the stone in the bath water and had no such reaction. It seems that there is no way to predict whether a reaction will occur or not.

One client, a good friend and staunch supporter of Essential Oil Therapy, called to report that she had a most unusual experience. She periodically goes to Arkansas to buy stones and has a wonderful collection. She had recently made a trip and purchased a remarkable set of stones that had formerly been the personal healing stones of a Native American medicine man. I saw the collection shortly after she purchased them.

One stone in particular was most unusual and powerful. It was a smoky quartz with other minerals in it colored red, deep forest green, and gold—a truly beautiful specimen.

The new owner of this stone decided that she would start her new bath series and substitute the smoky quartz healing stone for the stone in her formula. She placed the stone in the water and mixed in the vinegar and essential oils. Then she got into the tub and sank underneath the water, leaving only her nose out of the bath water.

Just as she was getting adjusted and comfortable, her eyes seemed to ignite. She shot out of the water and immediately ran to the sink and splashed cold water on her face and eyes. After a few minutes the burning stopped, and she took the healing stone out of her bath and replaced it with the stone in her formula. When she reentered the tub she completed her bath without any further discomfort. Fortunately, she had done numerous baths and had taken my introductory course. She understood what was happening and knew what to do.

Whenever there is burning of this nature, it always means that something in the energy field is being cleared. Burning around the eye area often indicates that thoughtforms over the eyes are disintegrating. Thoughtforms over the eyes are quite common, but in some cases stones that are substituted or added to the original formula amplify the energies in the water too intensely.

One of the steps in creating a personal bath formula for an individual is to check the person to see whether it is necessary to coat the skin with a vegetable oil and whether this oil also should be added to the water. If a powerful formula is needed in order to clear negative energies, the formula may or may not cause a burning sensation on the skin. If the person needs to protect the skin, then the appropriate oil, along with directions, becomes part of the formula.

Taking essential oil baths entails a step-by-step learning process for the client. The baths are not to be approached with a careless or cavalier attitude.

5

The Bathtub

The single most problematic aspect of successful Essential Oil Therapy is the bathtub of today. It is too short and too shallow for the average person. This is more true in apartments than in private homes. The ideal tub is the old porcelain clawfoot tub. It is deep and long enough to allow a tall man to relax comfortably. The majority of tubs today are no longer porcelain. Most of them are made of synthetic materials, and they do not have the lovely feel or shine that the porcelain tubs have.

The average bathtub, called a builder's tub, holds thirty-three gallons of water and measures fourteen inches by thirty inches by five feet. This is the tub generally found in moderately priced suburban homes. Most of the bathtubs in apartments are closer to four feet in length, which is the outside measurement. They are also more narrow and have less depth than the builder's tub.

We have become a nation of shower lovers, because the shower better suits today's hectic lifestyles. Many residences today have only showers. But in order to properly take an essential oil bath it is necessary to get all of the major chakras under water, and for this a bathtub is essential. The best positions are shown on page 81. One can move about, turning from side to side or lying on the stomach and dunking the head occasionally. The important thing is to get the head chakras under the water as much as possible.

The following precautions should be noted before essential oil baths are taken:

✧ Do not put essential oils in a Jacuzzi. They will clog the filtering system.

✧ Do not leave the bath water standing in the tub. Over a long period of time it will take the finish off of a porcelain tub.

✧ Do not use Epsom salts or sea salt mixed with an essential oil bath in a tub made of synthetic materials. The combination is too strong and is not even recommended for porcelain tubs.

For a deeper bath the overflow drain can be sealed. The best way to seal the drain depends on the kind of drain opening. Some are solid plates with slits around the sides. These are easy to seal. Take a small piece of cotton flannel and stuff the cloth into the slits with a knife. If the slits are tightly stuffed no water will escape.

Some tubs have an overflow drain that is a circular plate with slits on the face of the plate. This type is more difficult to seal. People have used different materials with varying success. Some people use putty; others use tape. Both are less desirable than a natural fabric. Any synthetic material in the water diminishes the effects of the bath to some degree.

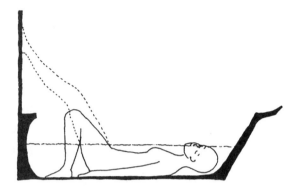

COMFORTABLE BODY POSITION IN BATHTUB
(FOR TALLER PEOPLE: LEGS EXTENDED WITH FEET AGAINST THE WALL)

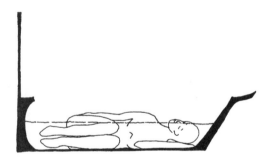

OPTIONAL BODY POSITION IN BATHTUB—WOMEN
(LYING ON SIDE WITH KNEES PULLED UP TO CHEST)

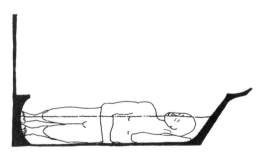

OPTIONAL BODY POSITION IN BATHTUB—MEN
(LYING ON SIDE WITH LOWER LEGS BENT)

Ideally you will have a nice big porcelain tub for your baths. If the tub is big and deep there is no need to plug the overflow drain, and you can lose yourself in the healing experience.

6

Bath Instructions
and Formulas

Essential oil baths require time and thought to prepare. At first the preparation process may seem too tedious and time-consuming, but after three or four baths the procedures become familiar and it gets much easier. Take the time, *make* the time, to get all the ingredients together and to organize everything.

Essential oils have different consistencies. The thicker oils are easier to count with droppers—but do not leave plastic droppers in the bottles. They will contaminate the essential oils, and the oils will warp them. Use a fresh dropper for each oil and do not mix them.

In the home, essential oils should be kept securely out of the reach of small children. Ingestion of these oils can cause serious damage—even death. Essential oils should be kept in a climate-controlled storage area and should not be exposed to heat above 90°F. The lids must be tightly sealed and the bottles stored away from sunlight in a dark, cool place.

Materials needed

- ⬦ Timer or alarm clock
- ⬦ Measuring cup
- ⬦ Wire whisk
- ⬦ A piece of cotton flannel, eight inches square

Optional:

- ⬦ Ear plugs
- ⬦ Snorkel
- ⬦ Candles
- ⬦ Pure, organic fruit juice
- ⬦ Tape player
- ⬦ Soothing or meditative tape

Ingredients for bath

- ⬦ Essential oil formula
- ⬦ Unprocessed apple cider vinegar
- ⬦ Stone designated in formula
- ⬦ Vegetable oil if specified

General directions

- ⬦ Allow thirty minutes to one hour to prepare for the bath emotionally, mentally, and spiritually.
- ⬦ Baths should be approached in an unhurried and meditative state.
- ⬦ It is preferable, but not required, to soap and shower prior to taking a bath.
- ⬦ The overflow drain should be plugged if the tub is shallow.

Preparing and entering the bath

- ⬦ Draw the bath, testing the temperature of the water. If it is too hot for you to submerge your face, adjust the temperature.

✧ If instructed in the formula, coat the entire body with the vegetable or fruit oil, paying special attention to the eyelids, face, and genitals.

✧ Place the stone designated in the formula in the bottom of the tub.

✧ Pour the measured vinegar into the bath water.

✧ Pour in the essential oil formula.

✧ Mix well with a wire whisk until no droplets are seen in the water.

✧ Pour in the vegetable or fruit oil if indicated.

✧ Mix well with the wire whisk.

✧ Do not step into the tub until the bath is drawn. The formula is for a minimum of thirty-three gallons.

✧ Use caution entering and exiting the tub if vegetable or fruit oil is used on the skin or placed in the water. Place a good nonslip rug by the tub to step onto when exiting. Sit on the edge of the tub and slide in, or roll over the edge of the tub. Slide down under the water, submerging the face and leaving the nose and a portion of the mouth out of the water. This position covers all the chakras and is the most effective. For comfort, turn from side to side or lie on the stomach, submerging the head frequently. It is important to keep the head submerged as much as possible.

✧ Tall people should sit up and soak their legs and feet an extra twenty or thirty minutes.

During the bath

Essential oil baths have a cleansing action that elicits physical, emotional, mental, and spiritual responses. The reaction to each bath is highly individualized, reflecting the family, heritage, childhood, lifestyle, temperament, personality, and past-life experience of the individual. Responses range from very subtle to very dramatic.

The two most common emotions to occur during the baths are anger and fear. These are the primary emotions that people repress to prevent being overwhelmed or losing control. People experience a gamut of emotional cleansing and clearings during the baths, including:

✧ Release of anger, fear, guilt, shame, sorrow, grief, anxiety, or depression
✧ Joy
✧ Deep relaxation
✧ Clarity and insight
✧ Past-life experiences
✧ Visitations and guidance from guides, angels, or relatives who have passed over
✧ Soul contact; being taken into the light and immersed in unconditional love

After the bath

✧ Block time to be alone and introspective.
✧ If one has high stress, fatigue, anxiety, worry, mental or emotional strain, or an illness, one's reaction to the first bath may be to fall into a deep sleep that lasts for twelve hours or more. Some people stay in bed for two days, sleeping deeply. This response allows all the healing energies to go into repairing any damage in the energy field.
✧ Do not shower or wash the hair unless absolutely necessary.
✧ A deeper connection with one's inner persona begins to develop.
✧ One's insight into life patterns begins to develop.

The release of pent-up emotions often results in a natural response: crying, yelling, pounding the tub, or a sense of relief as the heaviness, tension, and depression melts away. Occasionally the baths work at such a subtle level that it feels as if nothing has happened. These subtle changes are often noticed by family and friends. Fiery oils that elicit the release of anger may cause a burning or stinging sensation on the skin, which can begin mildly and then start to escalate. Often the stinging levels off just before it becomes too uncomfortable. It can stay at that level for up to twenty minutes and then suddenly it is gone. Should it continue to escalate, it is best to get out of the water and splash the face and warm body spots with cold water. If needed, another coating of the vegetable oil may be applied. Fiery oils that elicit the release of anger are allspice, bitter almond, cassia bark, cinnamon bark, cinnamon leaf, clove bud, garlic, ginger, onion, red thyme, and white thyme.

The milder oils for releasing and dissipating anger may create a stinging sensation also. They are Peru balsam, basil, juniper berry, sassafras, and tangerine.

If these oils are in a formula olive oil can be kept by the tub as a routine precaution to rub on the skin, should it be needed. It can also be added to the bath water one tablespoon at a time if needed.

The baths act on the physical body as developing solution does on photographic paper. Many clients have reported that strange-looking geometric markings show up on the skin. In some cases they are indicators of events from past lives.

In numerous cases people have reported identical matching welts appearing across the backs of both legs where as children they were struck with a belt or stick.

Sometimes a rash will break out in certain areas. This is a diffused release of anger and usually occurs with people who are soft-spoken and have a real aversion to their anger. This type of release is comparable to an energy mist, rising out of the body. Once the release is complete, all the skin reactions disappear.

An example of this reaction is the experience of a client who started taking the baths shortly after Essential Oil Therapy was launched. From the first bath this man had some profound experiences. His demeanor, his outlook, and the way he lived his life completely changed. He continued on a regular bath regimen, with periodic breaks, for several years and came to regard them as infallible guidelines for his life. He had received a great deal of insight into numerous past lives and how they affected many of his attitudes and talents in this life.

The client had recently begun a new bath series. He was working with a husband-and-wife team in rebirthing sessions and was getting dressed to go to a session when his entire body broke out in a rash. (This is by far the most extensive outbreak anyone has ever reported.)

Not panicking, he decided that his outbreak was in preparation for his rebirthing session. He had been working on releasing anger and had been stuck. When he got to the place where the water rebirthing was done, he put on his swimming trunks and got into the water. He and his counselors worked for three hours in the pool, releasing anger. When they were finished his rash was gone—completely gone.

Another recent incident happened with a client who had nearly completed her first bath series. She wanted to speak with me about her bath experiences and also needed an updated formula for her second series. When we met for our appointment, she told me that she was experiencing rashes in particular areas. Her hands and forearms had broken out with itchy red splotches, and from the knees down her legs had red splotches. As she spoke she extended both her hands. They were a solid bright red, extending past the wrists. A clear line at the same place on both hands marked where the redness ended and the skin became normal. There were random splotches on the forearms, and they also itched.

When the redness on her hands had begun to appear, she asked in the bath that she be given the information and understanding of why this was happening. Immediately she saw herself as a man in London in a past life. She had been caught and charged with rape. As punishment, both hands were chopped off.

In another bath she asked about her legs and received a glimpse of a fire where she had been badly burned on her legs.

The woman needed three formulas to address her situation. One was for a regular bath series. Another formula was for her hands, which needed to be soaked in a large basin, and the third was a sitz bath formula for her legs.

She continued to have small itching areas on her legs and stiffness in one knee. We temporarily stopped the baths, and she went back to a therapist who does energy work, to help unblock the energy. While he was working on her he asked what she had been doing, because her energy field looked so much better than when he had last seen her.

After several sessions her legs cleared up, but the knee was still bothering her. She called to say that she and her husband were going on a trip to Ireland and England with a group of friends. She was concerned about her ability to move about and wanted to see whether a new bath formula might help.

There were still layers of anger to be cleared, but because of her trip she needed to stop the releasing process of the baths. I deleted the anger oils and gave her a formula without them. She took the bath that night and said that it was very soothing and mild. Her knee felt much better; the pain and stiffness disappeared. She felt very good about the improvement and was relieved that she would be able to move with ease on her trip.

This woman has been exceptional in her ability to comprehend the significance of what was happening and to participate in getting her own answers. Even though some of the emotions from her past lives were restimulated, she was able to stay focused and centered. She exhibited a remarkable ability to step out of the situation, observe the energies at play, and persevere with a determination that is unusual.

Repressed anger is the underlying emotional cause of skin eruptions and the underlying emotional energy that sets up the breeding ground for cancer. Think about the chemicals and the radiation produced and put into our atmosphere. These energies are hostile to our very planet and contaminate the water, soil, and air. Anger is anger, regardless of the method or source from which it is projected.

As demonstrated by the previous examples, red splotches emerge on the skin where there are energy blockages. These are always areas where physical, emotional, or mental traumas or charged issues are stored. Noting the location of the markings on the skin can jolt the memory into recollection of specific, often forgotten events. This process is helpful in catalyzing a review and release.

People will respond differently to the same formula. For instance, some people are sensitive to the fiery oils and others not at all. The energies of each of our subtle bodies determine how we respond to any given formula. Each person is a complex mixture of a variety of specific energies, so each formula must be tailored to suit the strengths and weaknesses of an individual's energy field.

For example, cinnamon is the master essential oil for transmuting and releasing anger. A person with a strong energy field might be able to take a bath with fifty drops of cinnamon oil with no physical effects. Others might react to far fewer drops if their skin is not protected with a vegetable oil.

Such a case happened with a dentist who had a formula with fifty drops each of four or five of the most fiery essential oils, plus several others. The formula seemed much too strong. I checked it several times and it came out the same each time.

We spoke at length about the oils in his formula. I cautioned him about the intensity of the formula and advised him to be careful. I went over the entire procedure in detail, explaining all the steps to take and the variety of reactions that might occur. He was confident and unconcerned.

When we next met he was rather casual about his bath, stating that it had been extremely warm, as though he had gotten his bath water too hot. Other than that it was the only discomfort he experienced.

This man was made of powerful energy, which set up a strong field hard to penetrate. An energy field of this magnitude is not easy to influence. It would likely take a series of these powerful baths to pierce his armor.

People with less dominant energy fields would likely react to fewer drops of cinnamon, especially if they were in a weakened state or extremely fearful or highly emotional by nature.

Possible responses to the baths

⋄ Mild to profuse perspiration

⋄ Extreme relaxation, even sleep

⋄ The opening of a deeply meaningful dialogue with self

⋄ A sense of agitation and restlessness. People who have continually racing minds will react this way. It is resistance to quietude, reflection, and giving up control.

⋄ A buildup of emotional/mental intensity that makes it impossible to stay in the water

⋄ A feeling of weakness (caused by letting go of stress, tension, anxiety, etc.)

⋄ An elevated sense of well-being

⋄ A renewed sense of hope and happiness

⋄ Heightened sensitivity, discernment, and perception

Should a feeling of overwhelming heat and a sense of extreme intensity occur during the bath, it is best to get out of the tub for a period of time. Using a washcloth or hand towel, splash cold water on your face and body where necessary. If needed, apply more vegetable oil on the skin. Note and record the time spent in the tub.

Now is the time to take a break. Slip into a comfortable robe; pour a glass of pure fruit juice of your choice; put on a tape of bells, drums, chants, or nature sounds; and sit quietly in a comfortable chair. Slowly sip the fruit juice, savoring the heightened sense of taste you will experience.

Monitor your shifts in mood and energy level, and relax into a meditative, reflective state until the intensity has diminished and the heat dissipated. Then return to the bath, adding another coat of the vegetable or fruit oil if that is included in the formula.

The above procedure may be repeated as often as needed until the full amount of time has been spent in the bath water. It is very important to stay in the water for the amount of time stated in the instructions. One may stay in the bath as long as desired beyond the minimum time noted in the bath instructions. Hot water may be added as needed.

In rare cases, several days after the bath a localized rash or cluster of small eruptions may appear. Draw a bath with thirty to forty drops of wild chamomile essential oil. Dissolve a cup of white powdered clay and add to the water, mixing well. The combination is soothing and cooling and neutralizes itchy areas almost immediately. The combination can be made into a paste and rubbed on the skin as well. It is extremely effective in relieving any discomfort. Aloe vera gel is also very effective.

The process of clearing emotional and mental dross is not unlike clearing the physical body of toxins through fasting or a purifying diet. The reactions described regarding rashes and welts are extreme and not what most people experience. Familiarize yourself with the information in this book so that the appropriate response may be taken if needed.

Essential oil baths are not always pretty or pleasant experiences, but we must remember that the baths do not cause the negative energies to be there. They simply draw the energies out and break them up so that they can be released.

An important step in taking personal responsibility for our growth and expansion of consciousness is to come to the recognition that we all have intangible, invisible influences in our energy fields that wield enormous control in our lives. The most natural and universal fear is fear of the unknown. That fear will keep us frozen in place until we come to a point where we no longer are willing to be controlled by it.

People with medical problems and pregnant women should be extremely cautious about using essential oils. Lavender, tea tree, lemon, lime, peppermint, spearmint, vanilla, rosewood, amyris, angelica root, carrot seed, the chamomiles (wild, German, and Roman), eucalyptus, and helichrysum are all mild and soothing essential oils. Of these, lavender and the three chamomiles are the most calming and soothing. Nevertheless, baths and massages in this book are not recommended for pregnant women.

If onion or garlic essential oils are used

Both of these oils can linger for weeks, especially if there is an angry or hostile atmosphere in the home. If sexual abuse or incest is taking place or drugs are being used, the smell of garlic can be out of all proportion to the amount used. It can linger even longer than onion. It is a most curious experience to observe the way in which these two highly powerful cleansers work.

If one is on a bath regimen that calls for either of these oils, there is no need to walk through the days reeking of offensive odors. The following precautions may be taken:

⋄ Wash your hair immediately after the bath. Have enough freshly squeezed lemon or lime juice to saturate your hair. After shampooing, allow the juice to stay on your hair while working it in for about five minutes before rinsing. A fragrant cream rinse can then be used. If the odor lingers, repeat again the next day.

✧ Wash towels, sheets, and sleepwear separately. If you hang them outside, the fresh air and sunshine will remove the smell.

✧ To clear odors from the house, raise the window in the bathroom if there is one. Make a spray of lime, lemon, and ylang ylang or other preferred oils added to water, and spritz throughout the house. Or use an essential oil diffuser or electric potpourri.

✧ Chefs have long known an unusual method of deodorizing the skin from cooking odors such as onion and garlic. Industrial cookware stores and some hardware stores carry palm-sized stainless steel bars which will take away these odors when rubbed over wet skin and hair. Depending on body chemistry it works better for some than others. It usually sells for under eight dollars.

These suggestions are only for extreme cases. Many people have used onion and garlic with no big upsets in the household. People with relaxed attitudes have moved through their clearings with little turbulence. Others have experienced major upsets that go off like exploding volcanoes. It all depends on alcohol and drug use, addictive patterns, and the abuse that may have taken place in the lives of family members. It equally depends on whether individuals are dealing with issues or repressing them.

ADULT BATH FORMULAS

On the day that the first bath of a series is taken, mark all dates and information for future baths on a calendar.

Without a record to refer to, it is impossible to stay on schedule or keep accurate track of when or how many baths are left to complete the series.

Alcohol

✦ 30 drops each lavandin, lime
✦ 33 drops each laurel leaf, lemon, black pepper, spearmint
✦ 5 cups unprocessed apple cider vinegar

Stone: azurite
Time: 30 minutes

Do 10 baths spaced 7 days apart.

Then do an Entities bath series followed by an Aura Damage series.

When you have completed the three series, repeat the whole cycle once. It alleviates cravings.

Wait 5 months before repeating.

The results for alcoholics who truly want recovery and who stay on a committed essential oil bath/massage program are remarkable. An example is the following letter:

> I want to express my deepest gratitude for the information on healing. Thought I might take a minute to share with you what an impact it has made on my life.
>
> I am thirty-four years old and have had major problems with drug and alcohol abuse since my early teenage years. This abuse included addictions to heroin, cocaine, marijuana, and everything else I could get my hands on. Addiction to alcohol just came with the territory.
>
> After living with despair about ever giving my addiction up, your little blue book [*Essential Oil Healing*

Baths, self-published] came across my path. I had tried willpower too many times to know better.

I read the book and put it away and continued my normal course of destructive behavior, moving many times because of my inclination to run away from my problems.

I moved into an old house that had a huge bathtub. I was really hitting a very low point in my life and decided to give the bath on alcohol addiction a try. I also decided to go to an Alcoholics Anonymous group.

Although I'm still fairly new to recovery I have had a major healing. The craving for alcohol and drugs have almost completely vanished. The freedom I now feel is empowering.

My attention has now turned to repairing the damage I've done to my physical and subtle bodies. In recovery I have been listening to alcoholics and drug addicts who are sober but still having major cravings after long-term sobriety.

I feel so fortunate for the healing and only wish others could have the same experience.

If there is any way I could help pass on the wisdom you have shown me I would be a humble servant.

Keep up the great work! I can't thank you enough!

Shortly after I received the letter, this young man came to see me for a personal formula. I recently spoke with his sister, who says he is still sober and doing very well.

Alignment of Physical/Etheric Bodies

- ✧ 3 drops garlic
- ✧ 23 drops clove bud
- ✧ 30 drops each celery seed, peppermint, tangerine

✧ 5 cups unprocessed apple cider vinegar

Stone: lapis
Time: 35 minutes

Coat the body with rosehip oil.
Do 15 baths spaced 7 days apart.
This bath is for correcting misalignment that results from accidents, serious illness, poisoning, radiation exposure, etc. Initially, many adults could need this formula. Once alignment has been achieved, it should not be necessary to repeat unless other severe traumas are experienced.

Allergies

✧ 30 drops each sweet marjoram, rosemary, vetiver
✧ 38 drops each eucalyptus 80/85, spruce, sassafras
✧ 3 cups unprocessed apple cider vinegar

Stone: lapis
Time: 40 minutes

Coat the body with walnut oil. Add 1 tablespoon to the water.
Do 12 baths spaced 2 weeks apart.
Wait 6 months before repeating.

Anger

✧ 25 drops cassia bark
✧ 30 drops each nutmeg, vetiver, sassafras, tea tree
✧ 5 cups unprocessed apple cider vinegar

Stone: clear quartz crystal

Time: 40 minutes

꙳

Coat the body with peanut oil, paying special attention
to the eyes, face, and genitals.
Do 8 baths spaced 3 weeks apart.
Wait 5 months before repeating.

Anxiety/Worry

✧ 30 drops each summer savory, tangerine, ylang ylang
✧ 33 drops each elemi, white thyme
✧ 3 cups unprocessed apple cider vinegar

Stone: clear quartz crystal
Time: 40 minutes

꙳

Coat the body with walnut oil.
Do 8 baths spaced 12 days apart.
Wait 2 months before repeating.

Aura Damage

This formula is to be done after accidents or other situations that cause aura damage.

✧ 36 drops each eucalyptus 80/85, spearmint, vetiver
✧ 40 drops each atlas cedarwood, ylang ylang
✧ 3 cups unprocessed apple cider vinegar

Stone: lapis
Time: 40 minutes

꙳

Do 10 baths spaced 5 days apart. Then do an Entities
bath series.
Wait 3 months and repeat the cycle once.

Bruises

✧ 38 drops each cardamom seed, rosemary
✧ 43 drops each peppermint, pine, tea tree
✧ 6 cups unprocessed apple cider vinegar

Stone: clear quartz crystal
Time: 30 minutes

Do up to 7 consecutive daily baths as needed.

If the bruises or other injuries are caused by a sharp blow, the Aura Damage formula should be done every other day for 5 baths, alternating with the Bruises formula.

Change/Transition

✧ 36 drops each Siberian fir needle, tangerine
✧ 38 drops each wild marjoram, petitgrain, white thyme
✧ 3 cups unprocessed apple cider vinegar

Stone: sodalite
Time: 30 minutes

Coat the body with sesame seed oil.
Do 7 baths spaced 7 days apart.
Wait 2 months before repeating.
Use this bath for moves, job changes, divorce, deaths, etc.

Circulation

✧ 30 drops each atlas cedarwood, peppermint
✧ 33 drops each amyris, eucalyptus 80/85, sassafras
✧ 3 cups unprocessed apple cider vinegar

Stone: lapis

Time: 30 minutes

༺

Coat the body with pecan nut oil.
Do 15 baths spaced 12 days apart.
Wait 7 weeks before repeating.

Completion/The Ability to Follow Through

This is a three-stage process, which requires 3 formulas to be done in sequence as shown.

Formula 1

❖ 30 drops each aniseed, white camphor, ylang ylang
❖ 3 cups unprocessed apple cider vinegar

Stone: black obsidian
Time: 20 minutes

༺

Do 5 baths in 5 consecutive days.

Formula 2

❖ 30 drops each galbanum, tea tree
❖ 3 cups unprocessed apple cider vinegar

Stone: lapis
Time: 20 minutes

༺

Do 7 baths taken every other day.

Formula 3

❖ 30 drops each celery seed, helichrysum, ylang ylang
❖ 3 cups unprocessed apple cider vinegar

Stone: lapis
Time: 20 minutes

❧

Do 7 baths spaced 7 days apart.

Drug or alcohol residues, auric damage, and entities will prevent this series from being effective. These conditions must be cleared before the above formulas are used.

Courage/To Face Truth, Obstacles

⬩ 36 drops each sassafras, teatree
⬩ 38 drops each red cedarwood, elemi
⬩ 5 cups unprocessed apple cider vinegar

Stone: clear quartz crystal
Time: 30 minutes

❧

Do 7 baths spaced 7 days apart.
Use as needed when emergencies arise.

Depression

For best results, this is to be done in 2 stages.

Formula 1

⬩ 30 drops each white camphor, clove bud
⬩ 3 cups unprocessed apple cider vinegar

Stone: clear quartz crystal
Time: 20 minutes

❧

Coat the body with peanut oil.
Do 7 baths spaced 7 days apart.

Formula 2

⬩ 30 drops each sweet birch, grapefruit, myrtle

✧ 5 cups unprocessed apple cider vinegar

Stone: lapis
Time: 30 minutes

Do 10 baths spaced 5 days apart.
Wait 7 weeks before repeating.

Detoxification

✧ 30 drops each clove bud, patchouli, rosemary
✧ 33 drops each red cedarwood, Dalmatian sage, spruce
✧ 5 cups unprocessed apple cider vinegar

Stone: clear quartz crystal
Time: 40 minutes

Coat the body with pecan nut oil.
Do 10 baths spaced 2 weeks apart.
Alternate every other week with the Vitalizing and Toning formula.
Wait 10 weeks before repeating the cycle.

Drugs

For best results, this is to be done sequentially with 3 formulas.

Formula 1

✧ 5 drops garlic
✧ 38 drops eucalyptus 80/85
✧ 40 drops each atlas cedarwood, lavender
✧ 5 cups unprocessed apple cider vinegar

Stone: clear quartz crystal
Time: 40 minutes

Do 10 baths spaced 7 days apart.

Formula 2

⋄ 40 drops each bitter fennel, grapefruit, lavender,
  petitgrain
⋄ 4 cups unprocessed apple cider vinegar

Stone: clear quartz crystal
Time: 40 minutes

Do 5 baths spaced 5 days apart.

Formula 3

⋄ 30 drops each sweet basil, petitgrain, red thyme
⋄ 33 drops each atlas cedarwood, lavender
⋄ 5 cups unprocessed apple cider vinegar

Stone : lapis
Time: 30 minutes

Coat the body with walnut oil.
Do 7 baths spaced 7 days apart.
Wait 5 months before repeating the cycle.

With this formula, begin a regimen of exercise, fresh air, sunshine, and a highly nutritious diet. After you have completed this series, allow the integration, healing, and stabilization to take place. Get plenty of rest and give your bodies the support they need to heal and come to balance. No other formulas should be used during the 5-month interval. Unless there are cravings or other circumstances that warrant repetition, there is no need to repeat the cycle. The Vitalizing and Toning bath is recommended, and occasionally other supportive formulas may be used. Oils that heal aura damage and eject entities are in the three formulas, so there is no need to do either of these series afterward.

Enthusiasm for Life

    ✧ 35 drops each tolu balsam, peppermint, spearmint
    ✧ 38 drops each carrot seed, citronella, ginger
    ✧ 5 cups unprocessed apple cider vinegar

Stone: clear quartz crystal
Time: 30 minutes

Coat the body with olive oil.
Do 10 baths spaced 15 days apart.
Wait 7 weeks before repeating.

Entities

For best results, this is a 3-formula process.

Formula 1

    ✧ 40 drops each atlas cedarwood, lavender, clary sage
    ✧ 4 cups unprocessed apple cider vinegar

Stone: clear quartz crystal
Time: 30 minutes

Do 7 baths spaced 3 days apart.

Formula 2

    ✧ 30 drops amyris
    ✧ 33 drops sweet orange

✧ 38 drops sweet almond
✧ 40 drops each Peru balsam, summer savory
✧ 5 cups unprocessed apple cider vinegar

Stone: clear quartz crystal
Time: 20 minutes

Coat the body with olive oil.
Do 10 baths spaced 10 days apart.

Formula 3

✧ 30 drops each white camphor, eucalyptus 80/85
✧ 40 drops each tolu balsam, lavender
✧ 4 cups unprocessed apple cider vinegar

Stone: sodalite
Time: 20 minutes

Do 10 baths spaced 7 days apart.

Unless there is some form of trauma that would damage the aura, there should be no need to repeat this cycle.

Entities attached to the aura can wreak havoc in the life of the host and can affect the lives of family members in a dramatic way. Crazy, unpredictable, unexpected, and out-of-control things happen in worst-case scenarios.

It is important to call in the angelic kingdom and go through the ritual detailed at the end of chapter 1 of sending the entities into the light. Until the host is cleared, this ceremony may need to be done for as many as 7 consecutive baths before all the entities leave. Occasionally there will be an entity that is powerful and resistant to leaving, but normally they go within the first few baths. Most people have a sense of relief and lightness, and they feel it when all the entities have left. Through kinesiology—

the use of muscle testing, dowsing rods, or the pendulum—
one may determine whether any entities still remain.

Certain behavior patterns indicate that entities are attached and interfering. They are

- Sudden radical behavior changes
- Distractibility; often cannot listen or stay focused
- Poor judgment
- Personality changes in interest, activities, friends
- Trouble with clarity in understanding actions and
  motives of others
- Repeated breaches of appropriate behavior
- Inability to learn from mistakes
- Inability to recognize irrational or out-of-control
  behavior
- Emotional volatility and instability
- Absence of the ability to be self-aware or self-
  analytical
- Indiscriminate sexual behavior
- Entrenched addictions
- Deterioration of ethics
- Unreliability, irresponsibility
- Lack of care for the rights or feelings of others
- Complete focus on self and personal gratification
- Self-destructive and bizarre behavior
- Inaccessibility and remoteness
- Anger, temper tantrums, irrationality
- Antisocial, aggressive behavior

Drugs and alcohol so lower the light in the energy field
that it is possible for a person to be taken over. People can
be utterly foolhardy when it comes to drugs. Drugs are
the great deceivers; they lure with the promise of experiencing the pleasures of other dimensions. The experiences

are in some ways similar to what happens during advanced meditation. The difference is that with drugs, a person is projected in an unnatural and unhealthy way into other dimensions for which he or she is completely unprepared. There is no control. One minute the experience is lofty and beautiful, and the next minute it can become ugly or terrifying. Meditation provides a steady advancement in building understanding of these other realms, steady self-discipline, growing infusion of light into the subtle bodies, strengthening on all levels, and gradual expansion of the ability to reach higher planes. It becomes a natural, gradual unfoldment whereby, through deserving effort, one is allowed to visit higher regions in a safe and productive manner.

Remember that energy is impersonal. It strengthens what it touches. It is very unsafe for people to come into contact with these higher energies prematurely and without going through the natural processes. The strengthening of negative energies within the individual is what causes "bad trips" and the fall into a downward spiral where people find themselves in the lower regions of the astral realms. People little understand the dangers they open themselves to with alcohol and drugs. Of the two, drugs are the more dangerous because they so quickly cause addiction and so quickly insert a very dark energy into the aura—an energy that could be compared to slime. Everyone has known family or friends who behave in ways that are bewildering and inexplicable. Parents with several children who have been raised in a nurturing environment and have been given love, guidance, and ethical training may suddenly have one child who begins sneaking out at night, skipping school, gravitating to a wilder set of friends, getting in trouble with the law, stealing the keys to the car or getting pregnant.

It is a parent's nightmare for which this illogical, out-of-control behavior has no explanation. We speak here of a stable home situation as an example. In many other conditions and environments, the influences are so negative that young people are at high risk. These situations are more easily pinpointed. What people often don't understand is that middle- and upper-class homes can be hit with this kind of destructive behavior. Often parents don't have a clue about the source. Parents can be blamed for not teaching, disciplining, or providing love for their children when in fact they may be excellent parents who are at a loss about the situation or what to do about it.

If you are a parent whose child has become someone you no longer know, who no longer acts or responds as the person you raised, then you may be dealing with the results of damage in the aura and entities influencing your child.

Similar situations can occur in adults, and they too can begin to act very differently. Most adults don't get as derailed as teens and children do when this happens. There are so many variances in the way entities gain access and show themselves through behavior patterns that it is impossible to give a complete picture. I have worked with so many people who have entities that I have a second sense about them when they are present. Once one develops the sensitivity to entities, it is often possible to know they are there by engaging the eyes and looking deeply into them. It requires training and experience.

This is a vast and very important subject that deserves much more attention than it gets. It is the source of much misery and misunderstanding. In more desperate cases it causes suicide and suicidal impulses.

Recently a woman in major crisis came for a consultation. She presented a calm and reserved demeanor, which belied the turmoil beneath the surface.

As the consultation proceeded, the truth of her situation began to come to the surface. The oils in her formula indicated despair and sorrow. She felt that her life was out of control and falling apart. She was exhausted and had major auric damage and numerous entities. She said that her home was permeated with an unhealthy presence. Her eight-year-old son was frightened in the house and would not sleep alone in his room. He was threatening to run away from home, was constantly in trouble at school, and was routinely being sent home for behavioral problems.

Her husband had been abused as a child and harbored resentment and rage. He was emotionally abusing their son. After thirteen years of marriage he was having an affair, which threatened to break up the home.

The woman felt overwhelmed. She was in a weakened emotional state and in deep despair. The day before her appointment, she had been out looking for a poison to give to her son and then to herself. She said that her plan had been to first administer the poison to her son and be with him as he died, and then to take the poison herself. What prevented her was that she was looking for a quick and painless poison and had been unable to find one that she felt would fill that description.

While she was out looking, she came across some essential oils and was drawn to investigate. The woman who helped her recommended that she get a consultation for a personal formula, and she made an appointment. This is how providence works. After a two-hour session, this woman went away with formulas for herself, her son, and her husband, and she had a much better understanding of the situation and issues with which she was dealing.

Often people have some sense of the truth of things. This woman did, but she had no one to talk to and was reluctant to speak of the presence in her home because there is so much superstition, fear, and misunderstanding.

There is no way to adequately convey the radical improvement in appearance, behavior, and overall well-being that takes place when people begin to get cleared with the baths or even with massage. Entities are routed and sent to higher regions where they, too, can be healed.

Fatigue

- ✧ 30 drops each cypress, galbanum, summer savory
- ✧ 38 drops sweet almond
- ✧ 36 drops each carrot seed, tagetes (marigold)
- ✧ 3 cups unprocessed apple cider vinegar

Stone: lapis
Time: 30 minutes

Coat the body with rosehip oil.
Do 7 baths spaced 7 days apart.
Wait 7 weeks before repeating.

Fear

- ✧ 40 drops each clove bud, geranium, white thyme
- ✧ 6 cups unprocessed apple cider vinegar

Stone: clear quartz crystal
Time: 40 minutes

Coat the body with olive oil.

Do 7 baths spaced 7 days apart.
Wait 3 months before repeating.

Forgiveness of Self

- ✧ 26 drops ginger
- ✧ 30 drops each myrrh, vanilla
- ✧ 36 drops spearmint
- ✧ 4 cups unprocessed apple cider vinegar

Stone: sodalite
Time: 20 minutes

Coat the body with almond oil.
Do 10 baths spaced 7 days apart.
Wait 10 weeks before repeating.

Forgiveness of Others

- ✧ 30 drops each elemi, palmarosa, spearmint
- ✧ 4 cups unprocessed apple cider vinegar

Stone: lapis
Time: 35 minutes

Do 10 baths spaced 5 days apart.
Wait 10 weeks before repeating.

Grief/Sorrow

- ✧ 30 drops each sweet basil, ylang ylang
- ✧ 33 drops each patchouli, white thyme
- ✧ 36 drops tangerine
- ✧ 3 cups unprocessed apple cider vinegar

Stone: clear quartz crystal
Time: 30 minutes

Coat the body with almond oil.
Do up to 10 baths spaced 7 days apart.
This bath may be taken as needed.
If the full series is done, wait 7 weeks before repeating.

Guilt

✧ 30 drops each helichrysum, nutmeg
✧ 36 drops each lime, white thyme
✧ 5 cups apple cider vinegar

Stone: lapis
Time: 30 minutes

Coat the body with almond oil.
Do 10 baths spaced 10 days apart.
Wait 2 months before repeating.

Hyperactive

✧ 30 drops each juniper berry, nutmeg
✧ 38 drops each citronella, sandalwood, tea tree
✧ 6 cups unprocessed apple cider vinegar

Stone: clear quartz crystal
Time: 35 minutes

Coat the body with walnut oil.
Do 6 baths spaced 7 days apart.
Follow this series with an Aura Damage series. Wait 7
weeks before repeating.

Insect Bites

✧ 30 drops each grapefruit, ylang ylang
✧ 36 drops each lemongrass, spearmint
✧ 5 cups unprocessed apple cider vinegar

Stone: lapis
Time: 20 minutes

Coat the body with sesame seed oil.
This bath may be done for up to 5 consecutive days.
Wait for 7 days before repeating if 5 consecutive baths are taken.
1 or 2 baths with several days intermission may be taken frequently.

Insomnia

✧ 30 drops each tolu balsam, vetiver
✧ 33 drops each atlas cedarwood, petitgrain
✧ 36 drops geranium
✧ 4 cups unprocessed apple cider vinegar

Stone: azurite
Time: 30 minutes

Coat the body with sunflower oil. Do 7 baths for 7 consecutive days.
This bath may be done every 7 days thereafter, if needed.

Jealousy

✧ 30 drops each bergamot orange, petitgrain, ylang ylang

✧ 33 drops each sweet birch, summer savory
✧ 5 cups unprocessed apple cider vinegar

Stone: clear quartz crystal
Time: 30 minutes

Coat the body with rosehip oil.
Do 9 baths spaced 10 days apart.
Every 5 days alternate with the Love/Accept Self bath.
Wait 7 weeks before repeating.

Loneliness

✧ 20 drops clove bud
✧ 30 drops each eucalyptus 80/85, grapefruit, tea tree
✧ 33 drops lemongrass
✧ 7 cups unprocessed apple cider vinegar

Stone: clear quartz crystal
Time: 30 minutes

Coat the body with walnut oil.
Do 10 baths spaced 7 days apart.
Wait 5 weeks before repeating.

Love/Accept Self

✧ 30 drops tolu balsam
✧ 33 drops each clove bud, tangerine
✧ 38 drops valerian root
✧ 5 cups unprocessed apple cider vinegar

Stone: clear quartz crystal
Time: 20 minutes

⸙

Coat the body with jojoba oil.
Do 9 baths spaced 2 weeks apart.
Wait 9 weeks before repeating.

Mental Clarity

✧ 26 drops galbanum
✧ 30 drops each clove bud, lovage root, white thyme
✧ 36 drops each white camphor, petitgrain
✧ 4 cups unprocessed apple cider vinegar

Stone: lapis
Time: 20 minutes

⸙

Coat the body with walnut oil.
Do 5 baths spaced 12 days apart.
Wait 2 months before repeating series.

Mental Tension

✧ 30 drops each sweet basil, lavender, nutmeg,
   ylang ylang
✧ 36 drops each bitter almond, ravensara
✧ 40 drops cardamom seed
✧ 3 cups unprocessed apple cider vinegar

Stone: lapis
Time: 30 minutes

⸙

Coat the body with grapeseed oil.
Do 7 baths spaced 5 days apart.
Wait 3 months before repeating.

Nerves

❖ 30 drops wild chamomile (or 23 German or 17 Roman)
❖ 33 drops each lavender, palmarosa
❖ 36 drops frankincense
❖ 5 cups unprocessed apple cider vinegar

Stone: sodalite
Time: 35 minutes

Do 7 baths spaced 5 days apart.
Wait 3 weeks before repeating.
Wild chamomile is not always available. Sometimes German or Roman chamomile can be found, so they are listed as substitutes, although they are precious oils and more expensive.

Radiation

❖ 30 drops each clove bud, nutmeg, red thyme
❖ 35 drops each ginger, sweet orange, ylang ylang
❖ 38 drops white thyme
❖ 5 cups unprocessed apple cider vinegar

Stone: malachite/sodalite
Time: 40 minutes

Coat the body with sunflower oil.
Do 7 baths spaced 3 weeks apart. First week: Radiation bath. Second week: Aura Damage bath. Third week: no bath. Repeat the cycle 7 times.
Wait 5 weeks before repeating.
Radiation causes extensive damage in the human energy field. In order to heal the energy field, the effects of

the radiation must be neutralized. Then the holes, tears, and weakened areas can be healed and strengthened.

Even if the heavy metals that cause radiation are flushed out of the system and the physical body no longer manifests symptoms of illness, the subtle bodies are still damaged and this leads to weakness, a strain on the nervous system, a depletion of the immune system, and eventually chronic problems that cause serious illnesses or diseases. If the human energy field is not whole and healthy, it always manifests as illness in the physical body.

Has your child had multiple X rays or had body scans with medical equipment? Essential oil baths for radiation are one of the best preventive steps to take. Where there is exposure of any kind on a regular basis the baths should be taken regularly, along with a diet that includes spirulina, other sea vegetables, lecithin, magnesium, potassium, iron, and A, B-complex, C, and E vitamins. People must learn to take preventive measures to protect themselves and their families.

People who live near nuclear power plants should check to see whether the water used to cool the core of the reactor is being dumped into the river. If so, the soil downstream is being contaminated. This contamination will get into any crops being grown. In some areas city water has been contaminated because radioactive wastes were dumped into the sewers. Children and pregnant women who live near microwave towers or high-voltage wires should move or at least take preventive measures. We must take personal responsibility in this area because those in power have failed miserably.

Taken regularly, these baths can go a long way to protect people from radiation. With continued exposure only so much can be done. It is important to identify sources of exposure and to monitor these sources.

Regret

✧ 30 drops each carrot seed, coriander seed
✧ 38 drops each cardamom seed, lime, sandalwood
✧ 4 cups unprocessed apple cider vinegar

Stone: clear quartz crystal
Time: 30 minutes

Coat the body with walnut oil.
Do 10 baths spaced 7 days apart.
Wait 3 weeks before repeating.

Self-Blame

✧ 30 drops each nutmeg, summer savory, ylang ylang
✧ 36 drops each peppermint, tea tree
✧ 38 drops rosemary
✧ 5 cups unprocessed apple cider vinegar

Stone: lapis
Time: 30 minutes

Do 7 baths spaced 7 days apart.
Do an Aura Damage bath series (wait 7 days between series).
Next do the Forgiveness of Others series.
Follow this with a Forgiveness of Self series.
Wait 7 months before repeating the cycle.

Self-Worth

✧ 20 drops each sweet basil, lavender
✧ 28 drops each cumin, tangerine

✧ 30 drops each geranium, bitter orange

✧ 7 cups unprocessed apple cider vinegar

Stone: lapis

Time: 40 minutes

Do 7 baths spaced 3 weeks apart. First week: Self-Worth bath. Second week: Forgiveness of Self bath. Third week: Love/Accept Self bath.

Wait 5 months before repeating.

Sexual Abuse

✧ 30 drops each citronella, geranium, patchouli

✧ 33 drops each white camphor, lime

✧ 40 drops juniper berry

✧ 5 cups unprocessed apple cider vinegar

Stone: lapis

Time: 35 minutes

Coat the body with walnut oil.

Do 10 baths spaced 7 days apart.

Wait 7 weeks before repeating.

Skin Abrasions/Cuts/Wounds

✧ 30 drops spearmint

✧ 36 drops each tangerine, valerian root

✧ 38 drops each amyris, atlas cedarwood, spruce, tea tree

✧ 5 cups unprocessed apple cider vinegar

Stone: clear quartz crystal

Time: 30 minutes

~❧~

Coat the body with rosehip oil.

Do 10 baths spaced every other day.

Follow this with a Trauma bath series.

If the skin abrasions are minor, the Trauma series may not be necessary. This bath series is for healing skin damaged by accidents or surgery. Once the wound has begun to heal it hastens the healing process and assists in diminishing scars.

Sore, Stiff Muscles and Joints

For best results this is a three-formula process.

Formula 1

✧ 20 drops each grapefruit, oak moss, sassafras

✧ 30 drops each nutmeg, ravensara, vetiver

✧ 3 cups unprocessed apple cider vinegar

Stone: lapis
Time: 20 minutes

~❧~

Coat the body with peanut oil.

Do 5 baths spaced 7 days apart.

Formula 2

✧ 20 drops each tolu balsam, wild chamomile (or 17 German or 14 Roman), myrrh

✧ 23 drops cassia bark

✧ 3 cups unprocessed apple cider vinegar

Stone: sodalite
Time: 20 minutes

~❧~

Coat the body with walnut oil.
Do 3 baths spaced 5 days apart.

Formula 3

⋄ 30 drops each cumin, litsea cubeba, vetiver
⋄ 33 drops each eucalyptus 80/85, oak moss, peppermint
⋄ 36 drops sassafras
⋄ 5 cups unprocessed apple cider vinegar

Stone: lapis
Time: 35 minutes

Do 5 baths spaced 5 days apart.

These bath series are for chronic problems. The Detoxification or Vitalizing and Toning bath series can be used for stiffness and sore muscles and joints harmed by heavy exercise or minor accidents.

Stress

⋄ 20 drops white camphor
⋄ 30 drops each angelica root, carrot seed, peppermint, ylang ylang
⋄ 35 drops each lavender, tangerine
⋄ 6 cups unprocessed apple cider vinegar

Stone: azurite
Time: 30 minutes

Do 8 baths spaced 15 days apart.
Then do the Nerves bath series.
Wait 6 weeks before repeating.

Trauma

- ✧ 20 drops wild chamomile (or 16 German or 14 Roman)
- ✧ 30 drops each amyris, white camphor, damiana, vetiver, sassafras
- ✧ 36 drops each eucalyptus 80/85, lavender
- ✧ 5 cups unprocessed apple cider vinegar

Stone: lapis
Time: 30 minutes

Coat the body with almond oil.
Do 10 baths spaced 5 days apart.
Wait 7 weeks before repeating.

Unkind, Abusive Treatment—To Relieve Hurt

- ✧ 20 drops cinnamon leaf
- ✧ 25 drops each helichrysum, lemongrass
- ✧ 30 drops each dill weed, lemon eucalyptus, sweet fennel, lavender, peppermint, white thyme
- ✧ 36 drops geranium
- ✧ 7 cups unprocessed apple cider vinegar

Stone: clear quartz crystal
Time: 30 minutes

Coat the body with walnut oil.
Do 15 baths spaced 7 days apart.
Wait 3 months before repeating.
If there has been severe abuse, several series may need to be taken.

Vitalizing and Toning

- ✧ 20 drops each clove bud, tangerine
- ✧ 30 drops each amyris, carrot seed, peppermint, sassafras
- ✧ 33 drops oak moss
- ✧ 1 cup unprocessed apple cider vinegar

Stone: lapis
Time: 30 minutes

Coat the body with almond oil.
Do 4 baths spaced 5 days apart.
Wait 3 weeks before repeating.

Clearing Thoughtforms from the Eyes

One of the strangest, most unexpected forms of clearing to present itself in Essential Oil Therapy has been the revelation that we develop thoughtforms over our eyes, often as the result of childhood issues or drug use. A whole field of study in this area has not been touched yet. The first time I became aware of the subject was when I checked on a friend on a hunch one night. He was not a close friend, and it was unusual for me to go to his home except by appointment, but I kept thinking of him, and the urge to check on him didn't go away.

When I arrived he was in great discomfort. His left eye was infected, and the eyelid was granulated and scratching his eye with every blink. He had been treating it for several days, but it kept getting worse. Since he was a body worker and herbalist, he had many resources to find effective treatment, but nothing seemed to help.

Looking at his profile, I saw a cone-shaped energy field over his eye. I put several drops of essential oils in the palm of his hand and had him lean over and cup his hand tightly over the affected eye. He sat in this position for several minutes. When he removed the hand from his eye, he felt immediate relief. He could blink without pain. I left him with a formula, which he used for a day or two, and his eye began to heal immediately.

Because I have researched the spiritual dimension of the oils and know what they are for, my interpretation of the formula was that this was a thoughtform, created in early, formative years, which had to do with mother issues.

In another case an executive with a computer firm called to say he had been in misery for days with an eye infection. Although he had been to several doctors and had spent a large sum of money for medical treatment and prescriptions, he continued to get worse instead of better. Both eyes were red, swollen, and painful.

Again we used the method of placing a few drops of oil in the palm and cupping the hand over the opened eyes. (The person always bends over to keep the oils from running down the arms.) There was immediate lessening of the discomfort. He repeated the process, and his eyes cleared up in a day.

The formula this man called for indicated the source of the problem to be drug use, specifically marijuana, which he was using daily. A type of encrustation builds up in the energy field and puts a curtain between a person and reality.

The irony was that this person had been active and in a position of leadership in his local spiritual community. He was by nature very mentally oriented. Perhaps his indulgence was an escape into the world of feeling.

Even the milder drugs are harmful. Their effects are more subtle and difficult to distinguish.

Formula for Eyes

> ❖ 1 drop each laurel leaf, mandarin orange, peppermint, vetiver

Drop essential oils into the palm of one hand.

If both eyes are inflamed, place the hands together and turn them over so that the essential oils are transferred to the palm of the other hand.

Do not spread the oils to the outer edges of the hands.

Use care not to get essential oils on the face or in the eyes.

Bend over and cup one or both hands over the opened eyes.

Keep the eyes open and allow the fumes to enter the eyes.

Take the hands away occasionally and allow the eyes to clear.

Repeat this process several times and periodically over the next day or two.

The fumes may cause the eyes to water or even sting a little. The above formula should begin to relieve discomfort immediately. If not, a personal formula is called for.

7

Instructions and Formulas for Massage

Today there are many vegetable and fruit oils on the market. If essential oils are used for a massage, then a carrier oil must be chosen from the selection. Many, but not all, of the carrier oils available are listed below. Some of them can be found only in health food stores. These oils should be purchased only in a health food store anyway. Commercial vegetable and fruit oils are processed. Only unprocessed oils are to be used for these formulas. The oils are:

- ✧ Sweet almond
- ✧ Apricot kernel
- ✧ Avocado
- ✧ Castor
- ✧ Flaxseed
- ✧ Grapeseed
- ✧ Hazelnut
- ✧ Jojoba

✧ Kukui nut

✧ Macadamia nut

✧ Olive

✧ Peanut

✧ Pecan nut

✧ Pumpkin seed

✧ Rosehip

✧ Safflower

✧ Sesame seed

✧ Sunflower

✧ Walnut

✧ Wheat germ

An investigation of the Edgar Cayce writings provides some very interesting and informative reading on the healing properties of some of these oils.

Massage schools often teach students not to use more than one ounce of carrier oil on a client. They also normally use a carrier oil of a lighter consistency. Olive and peanut oil, for instance, are both heavier oils, but in an essential oil massage they work very well. For adults, two ounces of carrier oil should be mixed with the formula for each massage.

These massages may be done in the home by friends or family members as well as in a professional massage office. The therapeutic value is primarily in the healing properties of the essential oils. A professional massage is an added bonus, and if the therapist does good energy work, it further enhances the results.

People need touching. This is one of the most beneficial aspects of massage. Many elderly people are isolated. Often they are ill and physically unable to get in and out of bed, much less a tub. They may simply be too weak, in pain, or too stiff. All these conditions can be improved with the essential oil massages. They bring much relief and relaxation.

Some people are too fearful to take the baths and go through the process alone. They are less tense and anxious with someone else to help them move through their emotional processing, and massage provides the stabilizing element they desire.

People who have been sexually abused frequently cannot bear the intimacy of being touched by a therapist. The terror that sometimes comes up is very real. In these instances, a spouse or trusted family member might be appropriate.

People who are bedridden and recovering from long-term illnesses or accidents can experience real benefit from massage with essential oil formulas.

The formulas listed are general. There is no assurance that they may not be too strong for some people, though many will be quite comfortable and a few will find them not strong enough. If there is any discomfort with a topical burning sensation, all that is required is to adjust the formula by adding more of the selected vegetable oil to the skin and to the formula.

MASSAGE FORMULAS

Alcohol

- ✧ 3 drops onion
- ✧ 20 drops myrrh gum
- ✧ 22 drops each grapefruit, helichrysum, northwest lavender (grown in the United States)

✧ 23 drops each cypress, tagetes (marigold)

✧ 33 drops each sweet basil, red cedarwood, celery seed, eucalyptus, sweet fennel, lime, nutmeg, mandarin orange

Carrier oil: safflower

Do 5 massages spaced 8 days apart, followed by one Detoxification massage.

Wait sixty days before repeating the cycle.

Anger

✧ 3 drops onion

✧ 20 drops each allspice, bitter almond, eucalyptus, spruce

✧ 22 drops each grapefruit, pine, vanilla oleoresin

✧ 24 drops each lemon eucalyptus, patchouli, vetiver

Carrier oil: olive

Do 4 massages spaced 2 weeks apart, followed by one Forgiveness of Others massage.

Wait 2 months before repeating the cycle.

Anxiety/Worry

✧ 23 drops each celery seed, geranium (bourbon)

✧ 33 drops each ginger, spruce, sweet fennel

✧ 35 drops each helichrysum, myrtle

Carrier oil: olive

Do 8 massages spaced 7 days apart.

Wait 2 months before repeating the cycle.

Aura Damage

> ✧ 33 drops each sweet fennel, helichrysum, Dalmatian sage
> ✧ 38 drops each sweet birch, cardamom seed, elemi

Carrier oil: avocado

Do 7 massages spaced 7 days apart. This massage is needed once per month for 5 months thereafter.

The Entity Attachment massage should be alternated weekly with this one for a total of 12 massages.

Bruises

> ✧ 23 drops each allspice, wild chamomile
> ✧ 36 drops each mandarin orange, tagetes (marigold)
> ✧ 43 drops each cassia bark, geranium (bourbon)

Carrier oil: sesame seed

This massage may be done as required.

Change/Transition

> ✧ 33 drops each anise, rosemary
> ✧ 36 drops each wild chamomile, myrtle, red thyme
> ✧ 38 drops each lemon, tagetes

Carrier oil: sweet almond

When circumstances warrant, do 5 massages spaced 7 days apart.

Wait 2 months before repeating.

Circulation

- ✧ 33 drops each bitter almond, lime
- ✧ 36 drops each carrot seed, sweet fennel
- ✧ 38 drops each atlas cedarwood, lemon eucalyptus, peppermint

Carrier oil: peanut

Up to 10 massages may be done, spaced 5 days apart. Wait 6 months before repeating.

Depression

- ✧ 26 drops each litsea cubeba, mandarin orange, petitgrain
- ✧ 33 drops each cinnamon leaf, clove bud, rosemary

Carrier oil: sesame seed

Do 4 massages spaced 20 days apart.
The Self-love formula may be alternated with this formula every 10 days for a total of 4 massages each.
Wait 3 months before repeating.

Detoxification

- ✧ 20 drops each white camphor, lemon eucalyptus, patchouli, vetiver
- ✧ 23 drops each bitter almond, clove bud, grapefruit
- ✧ 25 drops each juniper berry, eucalyptus

Carrier oil: walnut

This massage may be done after an illness or recovery from an accident or hospitalization. Do 5 massages spaced 7 days apart or alternate with Nerves massage or Vitalizing/General Toning massage for a total of 5 to 15 massages. Wait 3 months before repeating this series.

Drugs

- ❖ 23 drops each sassafras, vanilla oleoresin
- ❖ 30 drops each geranium (bourbon), mandarin orange, palmarosa
- ❖ 40 drops each cardamom seed, lime, litsea cubeba, vetiver

Carrier oil: walnut

Do 7 massages spaced 5 days apart followed by 3 Detoxification massages.

Wait 3 months before repeating. Alleviates cravings.

For best results the body should be wrapped in hot towels soaked in unprocessed vinegar and water after the oils are applied.

Entity Attachment

- ❖ 30 drops each amyris, sweet birch, sassafras
- ❖ 33 drops each bitter almond, grapefruit, nutmeg
- ❖ 36 drops each atlas cedarwood, geranium (bourbon), lemon

Carrier oil: pecan nut or peanut

Do 5 massages spaced 2 weeks apart.

The visualization for calling in the angelic helpers to assist is critical. The massage therapist or person applying the essential oil formula can help by talking through the process.

Fatigue

- ❖ 20 drops each cardamom seed, citronella
- ❖ 23 drops each allspice, red cedarwood
- ❖ 25 drops each lemon, lime, vetiver
- ❖ 28 drops each atlas cedarwood, juniper berry

Carrier oil: rosehip

❧

Alternate Fatigue and Vitalizing/General Toning formulas for 5 massages each, spaced 7 days apart.
Wait 3 months before repeating.

Fear

- ❖ 30 drops each laurel leaf, nutmeg
- ❖ 33 drops aniseed
- ❖ 36 drops each tolu balsam, lemon, tea tree
- ❖ 38 drops each allspice, sassafras, vetiver

Carrier oil: sesame seed

❧

Fear and Trauma massages should be alternated at weekly intervals for a total of 12 massages.
Wait 6 months before repeating.

Forgiveness of Self

- ❖ 2 drops garlic
- ❖ 23 drops each bitter almond, carrot seed, atlas cedarwood, lemon eucalyptus, vetiver

Carrier oil: peanut

Do 5 massages spaced 2 weeks apart.
Wait 3 months before repeating.

Forgiveness of Others

✧ 28 drops each aniseed, helichrysum
✧ 30 drops each rosemary, spearmint, tea tree
✧ 33 drops each carrot seed, sweet fennel

Carrier oil: olive

Do 8 massages spaced 2 weeks apart.
Follow this with 4 each of the Grief/Sorrow and Anger massages alternately, in that order.
Wait 6 months to repeat.

Grief/Sorrow

✧ 22 drops lime
✧ 25 drops each eucalyptus, juniper berry
✧ 28 drops dill weed
✧ 33 drops each carrot seed, red cedarwood, tea tree

Carrier oil: peanut

Do 8 massages spaced 5 days apart.
Wait 3 months before repeating.

Insomnia

✧ 26 drops each eucalyptus, spruce
✧ 33 drops each lavandin, wild marjoram, vetiver
✧ 36 drops each aniseed, carrot seed, juniper berry

Carrier oil: walnut

This massage may be done as needed.

Nerves

- ✧ 20 drops each white camphor, lemongrass
- ✧ 26 drops each frankincense, spruce
- ✧ 23 drops each eucalyptus, spearmint, bergamot orange
- ✧ 30 drops each aniseed, celery seed, galbanum, geranium (bourbon), lavender, peppermint

Carrier oil: sesame seed.

Do 5 massages spaced 7 days apart.

This massage series may be done before or after the Drug, Alcohol, Fear, and Trauma series.

Radiation

- ✧ 3 drops onion
- ✧ 25 drops each lime, tea tree
- ✧ 30 drops each atlas cedarwood, cinnamon leaf, lemon, myrtle, peppermint, vetiver
- ✧ 33 drops each amyris, clove bud
- ✧ 36 drops each citronella, nutmeg
- ✧ 38 drops northwest lavender (grown in the United States)

Carrier oil: walnut

Do 3 massages spaced 2 weeks apart.

Wait 4 months before repeating.

This formula is for after exposure to radiation. It may

be followed by a weekly massage as needed with 25 drops each of bitter fennel and sweet orange.

Self-Worth

- ✧ 23 drops each citronella, geranium (bourbon), spearmint
- ✧ 33 drops each lavandin, lime
- ✧ 36 drops amyris
- ✧ 38 drops grapefruit

Carrier oil: sesame seed

Do 7 massages spaced 7 days apart.

May be repeated after 3 weeks if needed for up to 3 series; then wait 6 months before repeating.

Self-Love

- ✧ 26 drops each frankincense, lavandin
- ✧ 28 drops each amyris, atlas cedarwood, sweet orange
- ✧ 30 drops each caraway, lavandin

Carrier oil: rosehip

Do 10 massages spaced 7 days apart.

May be repeated after 3 weeks for up to 3 series; then wait 6 months before repeating.

Sexual Abuse

- ✧ 20 drops each bitter almond, sassafras, spruce
- ✧ 22 drops each sweet birch, cinnamon leaf, northwest

lavender (made in the United States), lemon
✧ 33 drops each helichrysum, litsea cubeba, mandarin
   orange, peppermint

Carrier oil: peanut

Do 5 massages alternated with 5 Forgiveness of Others
massages, spaced 7 days apart.
Wait 3 months before repeating.

Sore, Stiff Muscles and Joints

✧ 20 drops each geranium (bourbon), lemon, spearmint
✧ 24 drops each atlas cedarwood, cinnamon leaf,
   citronella
✧ 33 drops each celery seed, lemon eucalyptus, grapefruit

Carrier oil: walnut

Do 8 massages spaced 7 days apart.
Wait 7 weeks before repeating.

Stress

✧ 20 drops each aniseed, myrrh gum, nutmeg, Dalmatian
   sage, spearmint
✧ 22 drops each sweet birch, geranium (bourbon),
   juniper berry, rosemary
✧ 24 drops each cinnamon leaf, wild marjoram,
   petitgrain
✧ 25 drops each cypress, grapefruit, mandarin orange

Carrier oil: sweet almond

Do 4 massages spaced 2 weeks apart.

This series may be repeated once if needed, then wait 8 months before repeating.

Trauma

- ✧ 20 drops each cypress, myrrh gum, spearmint
- ✧ 26 drops each grapefruit, Dalmatian sage
- ✧ 36 drops each celery seed, eucalyptus, lemon eucalyptus, lavender, lemongrass

Carrier oil: avocado

Use to alleviate shock from old or recent physical, emotional, or mental trauma.

Do 4 massages spaced 2 weeks apart.

Repeat for extremely traumatic situations.

Normally wait 2 months before repeating.

Unkind/Abusive Treatment—To Relieve Hurt

- ✧ 2 drops onion
- ✧ 20 drops juniper berry
- ✧ 23 drops each lavender, rosemary
- ✧ 33 drops each bitter almond, amyris, eucalyptus, myrtle
- ✧ 36 drops each spike lavender, white thyme

Carrier oil: avocado

Do 7 massages spaced 2 weeks apart.

This series may be alternated weekly with one or both of the Forgiveness of Others or Grief/Sorrow series. Then wait 3 months before repeating.

Vitalizing/General Toning

- ✧ 20 drops each myrtle, spearmint, spruce
- ✧ 23 drops each eucalyptus, lavender, lemon, nutmeg
- ✧ 33 drops each allspice, davana, spike lavender, myrrh gum, rosemary

Carrier oil: walnut

Do 5 massages spaced 7 days apart.
Wait 4 weeks before repeating.

Caution: Do not get essential oils in the eyes while applying the massage mixtures. Essential oils will cause the eyes to burn. Should this happen, irrigate the eyes with cool water.

These guidelines for using the massage formulas are simply to maintain a reasonable pacing of the application of the formulas. Essential oils produce intense clearings and should be approached with respect and balanced usage.

Massages are an excellent way to introduce Essential Oil Therapy to those who are new to alternative healing practices. The healing hands of a trusted, knowledgeable therapist or the touch of a loved one is soothing and reassuring. Some people may prefer this route. Others may alternate baths with massages. For those who don't have tubs, an essential oil massage is the next best choice. The depth of relaxation is quite remarkable. Those who are lucky enough to have a trained Essential Oil Therapy practitioner who can mix a personalized formula will have an experience to remember.

Appendix A

List of Essential Oils

The list below may not be complete. Every company carries its own selection of essential oils. It is difficult to stay current because new oils are steadily introduced to the market.

For purposes of Essential Oil Therapy, the 1/3-ounce bottles should be the smallest size purchased. When there is a choice, organic essential oils are always recommended above nonorganic oils. Each oil is unique, not interchangeable as a substitute for another oil. Never substitute a similar-sounding oil for another.

The extraction process for sassafras does not remove all of the solids. Therefore, it is not considered a true essential oil because it is somewhat impure. But it is the only sassafras available, and since it is an important one, it is used in formulas.

ESSENTIAL OILS
(Oils in italics can also be obtained in organic grade)

Ajowan
Allspice berry (pimento)
Almond, Bitter
Amyris (candlewood)
Anise raven
Aniseed (anise)
Anise, Star (aniseed)
Artemisia, douglas
Balsam, copaiba
Balsam, Peru
Balsam, tolu
Basil, exotic
Basil, sweet french
Bay (rum)
Benzoin (absolute)
Birch, sweet
Cajeput
Calamus Root (sweet flag)
Camphor, white (camphor)
Caraway seed
Cardamon seed
Carrot seed (Queen
  Anne's lace)
Cassia bark
Cedar leaf, thuja
Cedarwood, atlas
Cedarwood, port orford
Cedarwood, red (juniper)
Cedarwood, Texas
  (juniper)

Celery seed (smallage)
Chamomile, Roman
Chamomile, wild
Cilantro, oregon
Cinnamon bark
Cinnamon leaf
Citronella
Clove bud
Coriander seed
Cumin
Cypress
Damiana
Davana
Dill seed
Dill weed, American
Elecampane (inula)
Elemi
Erigeron
Eromenth
Eucalyptus
Eucalyptus, lemon
Eucalyptus, peppermint
Fennel, bitter
Fennel, sweet
Fir needle, Canadian
Fir needle, Siberian
Fir needle, silver
Foraha (kamani tree)
Frankincense
Galbanum

Garlic
Geranium (bourbon)
Ginger
Gotukola
Grapefruit
Guaiawood
Helichrysum (immor-
telle)
Hop flowers
Hyssop
Juniper berry
Labdanum (cistus)
Laurel leaf (bay leaf)
Lavandin
Lavender
Lavender, northwest
Lavender, spike
Lemon
Lemongrass
Lime, pressed
Linaloe Wood (Indian
lavender)
Litsea cubeba (may
chang)
Lovage root
Marjoram, sweet
*Marjoram, wild (Spanish
thyme)*
Mentha citrata (lemon
mint)
Mugwort (wormwood)
Myrrh gum
Myrrh, sweet

Myrtle
Niaouli
Nutmeg
Oak Moss (absolute)
Onion
Orange, bergamot
Orange, bitter
Orange, mandarin
Orange, sweet
Oregano
Palmarosa
Parsley seed
Parsnip
Patchouli
Pennyroyal, American
Pennyroyal, European
Pepper, black
Pepper, green
Peppermint
Petitgrain (bigarde)
Pine
Pine, white (American)
Ravensara
Red mandarin
Rosemary
Rosewood
Rue
Sage, clary
Sage, clary (American)
Sage, dalmatian
Sandalwood
Sassafras
Sassafras, Brazilian

Savory, summer

Spearmint

Spikenard

Spruce

St. John's wort

Storax (Levant styrax)

Tagetes (marigold)

Tangerine

Tansy, wild

Tarragon

Tea tree

Therebentine (pinesap)

Thyme, red

Thyme, white

Turmeric

Valerian root

Vanilla, oleoresin

Verbena

Vetiver (bourbon)

Violet leaves

Wintergreen, American

Yarrow (milfoil)

Ylang ylang

PRECIOUS OILS

Angelica root

Chamomile, blue Egyptian

Chamomile, German

Jasmine (absolute)

Lotus, white

Melissa

Neroli

Rose (absolute)

Appendix B

Essential Oil Therapy Classes

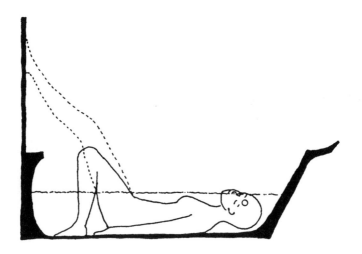

For information on how to obtain a personal consultation or class schedules for Essential Oil Therapy, contact me at the address below. If interested in the training class for professionals, please specify. Send a stamped, self-addressed envelope for replies via mail.

Milli D. Austin, P.O. Box 4778, Lago Vista, Texas 78645
Fax: 281-996-0138, Email: austin@gritman.com
Web page: http://www.gritman.com

Appendix C

Resources for Essential Oils

The most consistent frustration in developing Essential Oil Therapy has been finding a reliable supply of essential oils for clients. Ideally, health food stores and bookstores that carry books on essential oils would both stock a full selection. This has not been the case. The best place to look for essential oils is at your local health food store, but even in large cities the selection is often spotty.

Clients report that clerks often give misinformation because they are uninformed. They frequently do not know the difference between an essential oil and a fragrance. For this reason, and to make it easier to obtain the needed essential oils of good quality, the following resources are listed.

For those who live in small communities that may not have health food stores, or where the local stores do not carry the needed selection, the resource below provides retail service via the Internet, by phone, or by mail.

Gritman Corp.
P.O. Box 2009
Friendswood, Texas 77549
Phone: 888-474-8626 (toll free)
International: 281-996-8910
Fax: 281-996-0138
Email: sales@gritman.com
Web page: http://www.gritman.com

If your local health food store does not carry essential oils, the following wholesale distributors are reliable sources. Service, selection, and quality of the essential oils will vary somewhat. Some of the companies are very large and well established. They tend to have good quality control and a wide selection. Therefore, the oils are usually of a good grade. The larger companies can take up to two weeks for delivery and their prices tend to be higher. Some of the companies have a smaller selection but provide a high grade of essential oils at very reasonable prices. Others provide overnight service with no shipping charges for a modest minimum order. With some companies the quality of the essential oils will vary, and the essential oils are less costly. It is up to the buyer to investigate these differences and determine which best suit his or her needs. No one company carries a selection of all the oils.

Esssential Oil Wholesale Companies

Aura Cacia
P.O. Box 399
Weaverville, CA 96093
Fax: 916-623-2626
Phone: 800-437-3301

Frontier Herbs
Box 299
Norway, IA 52318
Fax: 800-717-4372
Phone: 800-669-3275

Hands-On AromaTherapy
for your BodyMind, Inc.
1558 Nanthalla Court
Atlanta, GA 30329
Phone: 800-331-6457
404-315-7010

New Concepts
P.O. Box 55068
Houston, TX 77055
Fax: 713-465-7106
Phone: 800-842-4807
713-465-7736

NOW Natural Foods
550 Mitchell Road
Glendale Hts., IL 60139
Fax: 630-545-9075
Phone: 630-545-9000

Starwest Botanicals, Inc.
11253 Trade Center Drive
Rancho Cordova, CA 95742
Fax: 916-638-8293
Phone: 800-800-4372
916-638-8100

Index

alcohol, 31-32, 107-108
  bath formula for,
    96-97
  massage formulas
    for, 129-130
allspice, 87, 130, 131,
  134, 140
almond, 112-113, 123-
  124
  bitter, 87, 116, 130,
    132-134, 137, 139
  sweet, 106, 111, 127,
    131, 138
aloe vera, 93
amethyst, 76
amyris, 100, 120, 123-
  124, 133, 136, 139
angelica root, 122
anise, 131
aniseed, 101, 134-136,
  138
apricot(s), kernel, 127
ashram(s), 2-3
astral body, 13-19
  diagrams of, 20, 28,
    31
astral plane, 13
attention deficit
  disorder, 32
aura, 9, 13
  damage of, 30-35, 45
  bath formula for,
    99
  massage formula
    for, 131
  ring-pass-not seal, 37

auric damage. *See*
    aura, damage of
autism, 32
avocado(s), 127, 131,
    139
azurite, 76, 96, 114, 122

balsam, Peru, 68, 87,
    106
  tolu, 105-106, 114, 115,
    121, 134
Barnett, Ann, 22
basil, 87
  sweet, 104, 112, 116,
    119, 130
bath formulas, 95-145
  alcohol, 96,
  alignment of bodies,
    97-98
  anxiety/worry, 99
  aura damage, 99
  bruises, 100
  change/transition,
    100
  circulation, 100-101
  courage, 102
  depression, 102-103
  detoxification, 103
  drugs, 103-105
  enthusiasm for life,
    105
  entities, 105-107
  fatigue, 111
  fear, 111-112
  forgiveness, of
    others, 112

  of self, 112
  grief/sorrow, 112-113
  guilt, 113
  hyperactive, 113
  insect bite(s), 114
  insomnia, 114
  jealousy, 114-115
  loneliness, 115
  love/accept self, 115-
    116
  mental clarity, 116
  mental tension, 116
  nerves, 117
  radiation, 117-118
  regret, 119
  self-blame, 119,
  self-worth, 119-120
  sexual abuse, 120,
  skin abrasions/cuts/
    wounds, 120-121
  sore, stiff muscles
    and joints, 121-122
  stress, 122
  trauma, 123
  unkind, abusive
    treatment—to
    relieve hurt, 123
  vitalizing and toning
    bathtub(s), 79-82
battering, 58
benzoin absolute, 69
Besant, Annie, 23-24
birch, sweet, 115, 131,
    133, 137-138
brow chakra. *See*
    chakra, ajna

Bruyere, Rosalyn, 57
Buddha, 11, 44

camphor, 65
  white, 101, 102, 106,
    116, 120, 122-123,
    132, 136
caraway, 137
cardamom seed, 100,
    116, 119, 131, 133-134
carrier oils, 127-128
carrot seed, 105, 111,
    119, 122, 124, 132,
    134-135
cassia bark, 87, 98, 121,
    131
castor, 127
Cayce, Edgar, 128
cedarwood, 99
  atlas, 100, 103-105,
    114, 120, 132-134,
    136-138
  red, 102, 103, 130,
    134-135
celery seed, 69, 97, 101,
    130, 136, 138-139
chakra (system), 8-9,
    43-62, 80
  ajna, 47-48, 57
    color(s) of, 48
    illustration of, 49
  crown, 28, 29, 32, 50,
    57
    color(s), of, 46-47
    illustration of, 46
    defined, 11
  hara, 58-60
  head, 57
  heart, 28-29, 49-51,
    58
    color(s) of, 51
    illustration, 50
  lung, 58
  medulla, 57
  root, 52, 53, 56-57, 58
    color(s) of, 57
    illustration of, 52
  sacral, 51-56, 57, 59
    color(s) of, 51
    illustration of, 52
  secondary, illustra-
    tions of, 59, 61, 62
  seven major,
    illustrations of, 54,

62
  solar plexus, 51, 57
    color(s) of, 51
    illustration of, 52
  spleen, 58-59
  throat, 48-49, 58, 59
    color(s) of, 49
    illustration of, 49
chamomile, 93
  German, 117, 121, 123
  Roman, 117, 121, 123
  wild, 117, 121, 123, 131
child abuse, 58
children, 32-35, 108-
    109, 118
chromosomes, 52
cinnamon, 68, 91
  bark, 87
  leaf, 87, 123, 132, 136-
    138
citrine, 76
citronella, 68, 105, 120,
    134, 136-138
clay, 93
clove bud, 87, 97, 102,
    103, 111, 115, 116, 117,
    124, 132, 136
coriander seed, 119
crown chakra. See
  chakra, crown
crystal, quartz. See
  quartz crystal
cumin, 119, 122
cypress, 111, 130, 138-
    139

damiana, 123
davana, 140
deva(s), 40-41
diet, purifying, 93
dill weed, 123, 135
drugs, 31-32, 107-108
  bath formulas for,
    103-104
  massage formula
    for, 133

elemi, 99, 102, 112, 131
emerald, 76
entities, 35-37, 40-41,
    96, 107-111
  bath formulas for,
    105-107
  massage formula

for, 133-134
Essential Oil Healing
  Baths, 97
essential oil(s), 1-2, 4-6,
    8, 9, 10, 27, 34, 38,
    43, 44, 60
  as antiseptics, 67
  and bathing, 64-65,
    70, 79-140
  and douches, 71-72
  extraction of, 64
  formula for eyes, 126
  healing properties
    of, 63-73
  and massage, 127-
    140
  storage of, 83
  and surgery, 69
etheric body, 10-13, 45
  alignment, 97
  diagrams of, 12, 20,
    28, 31
  viewing of, 12-13
eucalyptus, 65, 98-100,
    103, 106, 115, 122-123,
    130, 132, 135-136,
    139-140
lemon, 123, 130, 132,
    134, 138, 140
eyes, 124-126

Farenthold, Sissy, 15
fasting, 93
fatigue, 11
fennel, bitter, 104
  sweet, 123, 130-132,
    135
fetal alcohol syn-
    drome, 34
fiery oils, 87, 91
fir needle, Siberian,
    100
flaxseed, 127
fluoride, 75
fluorite, purple, 76
frankincense, 117, 136-
    137

galbanum, 101, 111, 136
garlic, 66, 87, 94-95,
    97, 134
garnet, 76
gemstones, 74-78
geranium, 114, 120,

123, 131, 133, 136-138
ginger, 105, 112, 117,
  130
Godforce, the, 18
grapefruit, 104, 114,
  115, 121, 129-130,
  132-133, 137-139
grapeseed, 116, 127

hara chakra. *See*
  chakra, hara
hazelnut(s), 127
head chakra. *See*
  chakra, head
heart, 58
  chakra. *See* chakra,
  heart
helichrysum, 101, 113,
  123, 129-131, 135, 138
herbs, 9-10
hyperactivity, 32

insect bites, 67-69, 114
integrated personality,
  25-27
intuition, 47
iron, 75, 118

jade, 76
Jesus, 44
jojoba, 116, 127
juniper berry, 87, 113,
  120, 132, 134-135,
  138-139

kinesiology, 68, 106-
  107
kukui, 128
kundalini, 25-26, 30
  rising of, 29

lamas (Tibetan), 29
lapis, 76, 98, 99-101, 103,
  111-114, 116, 119-124
laurel, leaf, 126, 134
lavandin, 96, 135, 137
lavender, 65, 103-106,
  116-117, 119, 122-123,
  136, 139-140
  northwest, 129, 136-
  138
  spike, 139-140
lecithin, 118
lemon, 96, 131-135, 138,

140
juice, 94
lemongrass, 114, 115,
  123, 136, 139
lime, 69, 96, 119, 120,
  130, 133-137
  juice, 94
litsea cubeba, 122, 132-
  133, 138
logos body, 30
  diagram of, 31
lotus, 45
lovage root, 116
lung chakra. *See*
  chakra, lung

macadamia, 128
magnesium, 75, 118
malachite, 76, 117
marigold. *See* tagetes
marjoram, sweet, 98
  wild, 100, 135, 138
massage formulas,
  127-140
  alcohol, 129-130
  anger, 130
  anxiety/worry, 130-
  131
  aura damage, 131
  bruises, 131
  change/transition,
  131
  circulation, 132
  depression, 132
  detoxification, 132
  drugs, 133
  entity attachment,
  133-134
  fatigue, 134
  fear, 134
  forgiveness, of
  others, 135
  of self, 134-135
  grief/sorrow, 135
  insomnia, 135-136
  nerves, 136
  radiation, 136-137
  self-worth, 137
  self-love, 137
  sexual abuse, 137-
  138
  sore, stiff muscles
  and joints, 138
  stress, 138-139

trauma, 139
  relieve hurt, 139
  vitalizing/general
  toning, 140
matrix (stone), 76
medulla chakra. *See*
  chakra, medulla
menstrual-cycle
  trouble, 56
mental body, 19-21
  diagrams of, 20, 28
mental retardation, 32
meridians, 11
minerals, 75
Mohammed, 44
monad body, 30
  diagram of, 31
myrrh, 112, 121
  gum, 129, 138-140
myrtle, 130-131, 136-
  140

nadis, 11
nutmeg, 98, 116, 117,
  119, 121, 130, 133-134,
  136, 138, 140

oak moss, 121, 122, 124
obsidian, black, 76, 101
olive(s), 105-106, 111,
  128, 130, 135
onion, 66, 87, 94-96,
  129, 136, 139
orange(s), bergamot,
  114, 136
  bitter, 120
  mandarin, 126, 130-
  133, 138
  sweet, 117, 137
ovaries, 49, 52, 56
ozone layer, 37

palmarosa, 112, 117, 133
pancreas, 51
patchouli, 65, 103, 112,
  120, 130, 132
peanut(s), 102, 121, 128,
  132-133, 135, 138
pecan(s), 101, 103, 128,
  133
pepper, black, 69, 96
peppermint, 97, 100,
  105, 119, 122-124,
  126, 132, 136, 138

peridot, 76
petitgrain, 100, 104,
    114, 116, 132, 138
pH balance, 75
phosphorus, 75
physical body, 10
    alignment, 97-98
    diagrams of, 12, 20, 28
pine, 100, 130
pineal gland, 48, 57
pituitary gland, 45, 48,
    57
plants, 39, 63
potassium, 75, 118
prostate, 56
pumpkin, 128

quartz crystal, 74, 75-
    76, 99
    clear, 76, 100, 103-
    106, 111, 113, 115,
    119-121, 123
    rose, 76
    smoky, 77

radiation, 117-118
ravensara, 116, 121
rebirthing (sessions), 88
redemption of matter,
    26
root chakra. See
    chakra, root
rosehip, 9, 111, 115, 121,
    128, 134, 137
rosemary, 65, 98, 100,
    103, 119, 133, 139-140
ruby, 76

sacral chakra. See
    chakra, sacral
safflower, 130
sage, clary, 105
    Dalmatian, 103, 131,
    138-139
sandalwood, 113, 119
sapphire, blue, 76
sassafras, 87, 98, 100,
    102, 121-124, 133-
    134, 137

savory, summer, 99,
    106, 111, 115, 119
scrotum, 52
sesame seed, 100, 114,
    128, 131-132, 134,
    136-137
sex, 51, 56
silicon, 75
smoking, 32
snake bites, 67-68
sodalite, 100, 106, 112,
    117, 121
sodium, 75
solar plexus chakra.
    See chakra, solar
    plexus
soul body, 27-30
soul, the, 48
spearmint, 96, 99, 105,
    112, 114, 120, 135-140
spine, the, 24, 45-47,
    53, 56
spirulina, 118
spleen chakra. See
    chakra, spleen
spruce, 98, 103, 120,
    130, 135, 137, 140
stomach, 51
subtle bodies, 7-42, 43.
    See also astral body;
    etheric body; logos
    body; mental body;
    monad body; soul
    body
    diagrams of, 12, 20, 28
    and radiation, 118
sugilite, 76
sulfur, 75
sunflower, 114, 117, 128

tagetes, 111, 130-131
tangerine, 97, 99, 100,
    112, 115, 119, 122, 124
tea tree, 65, 98, 100-102,
    113, 115, 120, 135-136
telepathic abilities, 47
testes, 52, 56
Theosophical Society,
    23-24

Thoughtforms, 23-24
throat chakra, See
    chakra, throat
thyme, red, 87, 104,
    117, 131
    white, 87, 99-100,
    111-113, 116-117, 123,
    139
thymus, 50, 58
topaz, 76
Tourette's syndrome,
    32
tourmaline, 76

University of Texas,
    14-15
uterus, 49

valerian root, 115, 120
vanilla, 112
    oleoresin, 130, 133
vetiver, 98, 99, 114, 121,
    122-123, 126, 130,
    132-136
vinegar (apple cider),
    69, 74-78, 96, 98-
    106, 111-117, 119-124
vitamin(s), A, 118
    B-complex, 118
    C, 118
    E, 118

walnut, 99, 113, 115-116,
    120, 122-123, 128,
    132-133, 136, 138, 140
watery plane. See astral
    plane
wheat germ, 128
Wheels of Light, 57

X rays, 118

yang, 53
yin, 53
ylang ylang, 99, 101, 112,
    114, 116-117, 119, 122
yoga, 1, 3-4